EMERGENCY OPHTHALMOLOGY

A RAPID TREATMENT GUIDE

NOTICE

Medicine is an ever-changing science. As new research and clini-cal experience broaden our knowledge, changes in treatment and drug therapy are required. The author and the publisher of this work have checked with sources believed to be reliable in their efforts to provide information that is complete and generally in accord with the standards accepted at the time of publication. However, in view of the possibility of human error or changes in medical sciences, neither the author nor the publisher nor any other party who has been involved in the preparation or publication of this work warrants that the information contained herein is in every respect accurate or complete, and they disclaim all responsibility for any errors or omissions or for the results obtained from use of the information contained in this work. Readers are encouraged to confirm the information contained herein with other sources. For example and in particular, readers are advised to check the product information sheet included in the package of each drug they plan to administer to be certain that the information contained in this work is accurate and that changes have not been made in the rec-ommended dose or in the contraindications for administration. This recommendation is of particular importance in connection with new or infrequently used drugs.

EMERGENCY OPHTHALMOLOGY

A RAPID TREATMENT GUIDE

Kenneth C. Chern, MD

Assistant Professor of Ophthalmology
Boston University School of Medicine
Boston, Massachusetts

McGRAW-HILL
Medical Publishing Division

New York   Chicago   San Francisco   Lisbon   London   Madrid   Mexico City
Milan   New Delhi   San Juan   Seoul   Singapore   Sydney   Toronto

McGraw-Hill

A Division of The **McGraw·Hill** *Companies*

Emergency Ophthalmology: A Rapid Treatment Guide

1234567890 IMA IMA 098765432

ISBN 0-07-137325-X

This book was set in Times Roman by Progressive Information Technologies.
The editors were Darlene Cooke, Susan Noujaim, and Karen Davis.
The production supervisor was Catherine Saggese.
The text designer was Marsha Cohen/Parallelogram.
The cover designer was Aimée Nordin
The index was prepared by Editorial Services, Maria Coughlin.
Imago, Singapore, was printer and binder.

This book is printed on acid-free paper.

Library of Congress Cataloging-in-Publication Data
Emergency ophthalmology / [edited by] Kenneth C. Chern.
    p. ; cm.
  Includes bibliographical references and index.
  ISBN 0-07-137325-X
  1. Ophthalmologic emergencies.   I. Chern, Kenneth C.
  [DNLM: 1. Eye Diseases–diagnosis.   2. Eye Diseases–therapy.
  3. Emergencies.   4. Eye Injuries.   WW 140 E53 2003]
RE48 .E445 2003
617.7'026–dc21   2001057900

CONTENTS

Contributors / ix
Preface / xi
Acknowledgments / xiii

1. ANATOMY   1

Scott M. Damrauer/Sudhir R. Vora

Anatomy of the Eye and Orbit / 1
    Adenexa / 1
    Anterior Segment / 6
    Posterior Segment / 10

2. BASIC EYE EXAMINATION   15

Sudhir R. Vora/Scott M. Damrauer

Checking Vision / 15
Visual Fields Testing / 20
Pupillary Examination / 23
Motility Examination / 26
External Examination / 27
Slit Lamp Examination / 30
Intraocular Pressure / 32
Funduscopy / 36
Color Vision Testing / 40
Stereoacuity Testing / 41

3. TRAUMA   43

Lauren Shatz/Corina Stancey

Corneal Foreign Body / 43
Corneal Abrasion / 46
Recurrent Erosion Syndrome / 50
Conjunctival and Corneal Laceration / 50
Chemical and Thermal Injury / 55

Hyphema / 59
Lens Subluxation or Dislocation / 62
Intraocular Foreign Body (IOFB) / 65
Traumatic Retinal Damage / 68
Ruptured Globe and Scleral Rupture / 72
Traumatic Optic Neuropathy (TON) / 75
Lid Laceration / 76
Blow-Out Fractures / 81

4. CONJUNCTIVA   85

Kambiz Negahban

Bacterial Conjunctivitis / 85
Viral Conjunctivitis / 88
Allergic Conjunctivitis / 92
Subconjunctival Hemorrhage / 95

5. CORNEA   97

Kambiz Negahban

Corneal Infections / 97
Contact Lens Keratitis and Infection / 102
Herpetic Keratitis / 106
Exposure Keratopathy / 110
Dry Eyes (Keratoconjunctivitis Sicca) / 113

6. UVEITIS   119

Kenneth C. Chern

Iridocyclitis and Traumatic Iritis / 119
Scleritis / 122
Endophthalmitis / 124

7. LENS   129

Kenneth C. Chern

Cataract Formation / 129

8. GLAUCOMA   135

Rohit Krishna/Michael Cassell

Angle Closure Glaucoma / 135
Hyphema and Traumatic Glaucoma / 138
Bleb-Associated Infections / 142
Phacolytic Glaucoma / 145
Neovascular Glaucoma / 148
Pseudoexfoliation Syndrome / 150
Pigmentary Glaucoma / 152
Steroid-Induced Glaucoma / 154

9. RETINA AND VITREOUS   155

Rashid Taher/Andrew Woldorf

Flashes and Floaters / 155
Vitreous Hemorrhage / 159
Retinal Detachment / 162
Diabetic Retinopathy / 168
Central Retinal Artery Occlusion and
    Branch Retinal Artery Occlusion / 173
Central Retinal Vein Occlusion and
    Branch Retinal Vein Occlusion / 176
Age-Related Macular Degeneration / 180
Macular Holes / 183

10. ORBIT AND PLASTICS   187

Corina Stancey/Susan Tucker

Contact Dermatitis / 187
Preseptal Cellulitis / 190
Orbital Cellulitis / 192
Chalazion and Stye / 196
Skin Cancers / 198
Dacryocystitis / 204
Proptosis / 206
Carotid-Cavernous Sinus Fistula / 210

11. NEUROOPHTHALMOLOGY   215

Jack A. Zamora

Visual Field Loss / 215
Double Vision / 219
Optic Neuritis / 220
Papilledema / 222
Pseudotumor Cerebri / 224
Anterior Ischemic Optic Neuropathy / 226
Cranial Nerve Palsy / 227
Myasthenia Gravis / 230
Abnormal Pupils and Anisocoria / 231
Afferent Pupillary Defect / 233
Migraine Headache / 234

12. PEDIATRICS OPHTHALMOLOGY   237

Melanie Anne Kazlas/Kailenn Tsao

Special Considerations / 237
Strabismus / 241
Leukocoria (White Pupil) / 244
Nasolacrimal Duct Obstruction / 247
Congenital Glaucoma / 250
Shaken Baby Syndrome / 254

APPENDICES

257

Scott M. Damrauer/Sudhir R. Vora

Appendix A: Amsler Grid / 258
Appendix B: Seidel Test / 261
Appendix C: Common Ophthalmic Medications / 263
Appendix D: Common Ophthalmic Abbreviations / 267

INDEX

271

CONTRIBUTORS

Michael Cassell, MD
Chief Resident, Ophthalmology
Eye Foundation of Kansas City
University of Missouri-Kansas City
    School of Medicine
Kansas City, Missouri

Kenneth C. Chern, MD
Assistant Professor of Ophthalmology
Boston University School of Medicine
Boston, Massachusetts

Scott M. Damrauer, BA
Student
Harvard Medical School
Boston, Massachusetts

Melanie Anne Kazlas, MD
Assistant Professor of Ophthalmology
Boston University School of Medicine
Boston, Massachusetts

Rohit Krishna, MD
Clinical Assistant Professor of Ophthalmology
Director, Glaucoma Department
Eye Foundation of Kansas City
University of Missouri-Kansas City
    School of Medicine
Kansas City, Missouri

Kambiz Negahban, MD
Department of Ophthalmology
Boston University School of Medicine
Boston, Massachusetts

Lauren Shatz, MD
Ophthalmology Resident
Boston Medical Center
Boston, Massachusetts

Corina Stancey, MD
Ophthalmology Resident
Boston Medical Center
Boston, Massachusetts

Rashid Taher, MD
Retina Fellow
Department of Ophthalmology
Boston University School of Medicine
Boston, Massachusetts

Kailenn Tsao, MD
Assistant Professor of Ophthalmology
Boston University School of Medicine
Boston, Massachusetts

Susan Tucker, MD
Lahey Clinic
Burlington, Massachusetts

Sudhir R. Vora, BA
Student
Harvard Medical School
Boston, Massachusetts

Andrew Woldorf, MD
Retina Fellow
Department of Ophthalmology
Boston University School of Medicine
Boston, Massachusetts

Jack A. Zamora, MD
Department of Ophthalmology
Boston University School of Medicine
Boston, Massachusetts

PREFACE

Prompt diagnosis and appropriate treatment are critical in ophthalmic emergencies to best preserve the integrity of the globe and vision in the eye. Prioritizing the differential diagnoses is a challenging task especially with overlapping signs and symptoms of many eye conditions. This book is designed for the practitioner to use in conjunction with the patient evaluation in the clinic or emergency room. The book highlights critical examination features and outlines initial treatment measures and follow-up guidelines for many common entities that present acutely.

The first chapter is an overview of the anatomy and structures in and around the eye. The second chapter describes the elements of the ophthalmic examination. The remainder of the book is organized by the predominant structure of the eye that is involved. Each disease is distilled into the key presenting features on clinical history and examination, treatment and follow-up outlines, and helpful ophthalmologic pearls.

KENNETH C. CHERN, MD

ACKNOWLEDGMENTS

With a book such as this, there are numerous authors to whom I owe a debt of gratitude for their scholarly work, excellent illustrations, and contributions to the body of ophthalmic knowledge. Many thanks to our friends and families whose continual support often goes unrecognized.

EMERGENCY OPHTHALMOLOGY

A RAPID TREATMENT GUIDE

Chapter 1

ANATOMY

SCOTT M. DAMRAUER
SUDHIR R. VORA

ANATOMY OF THE EYE AND ORBIT

The eye and its associated structures (Fig. 1-1) can be divided into six separate anatomical divisions: (1) adnexa, consisting of the eyelids and lacrimal apparatus; (2) anterior segment, composed of the conjunctiva, cornea, and anterior chamber; (3) iris and lens; (4) posterior segment, consisting of the vitreous, retina, choroid, and sclera; (5) extraocular muscles; and (6) orbit. Each segment contains a number of structures that are both anatomically and functionally related.

ADENEXA

EYELIDS The eyelids serve to protect the eyes from the environmental injury and trauma and to keep the ocular surface moist by both preventing evaporative drying of the conjunctiva and cornea and helping to spread tears produced by the lacrimal glands. The eyelids consist of five layers of tissue (Fig. 1-2), from superficial to deep: the skin, a muscular layer (orbicularis oculi muscles), a layer of loose areolar connective tissue, a fibrous layer (the tarsus), and an internal mucous membrane (the conjunctiva). When open, the elliptical space between the lid margins is referred to as the palpebral fissure and extends from the lateral canthus on the temporal side of the eye, to the medial canthus on the nasal side of eye. Adjacent to the medial canthus is the caruncle, a small yellowish structure that consists of modified sweat and sebaceous glands and the plica semilunaris, a vestigial remnant of the third eyelid formed by a folding of the conjunctiva.

Located in the margin of the eyelid between the fibrous layer and internal mucous membrane are the meibomian glands, which secrete sebum into the tear fluid. Also located along the eyelid margin are the hair follicles of the eyelashes. The sebaceous glands of Zeis and the sweat glands of Moll are adjacent to the hair follicles.

The lids receive blood from branches of both the lacrimal and ophthalmic arteries, and drain to the ophthalmic veins and the veins draining the forehead. Lymphatic drainage from the medial aspect of the lids goes to the submandibular nodes, while that from the lateral aspect drains to the preauricular and parotid nodes. The upper eyelid is innervated by CN V_1 and the lower eyelid by CN V_2.

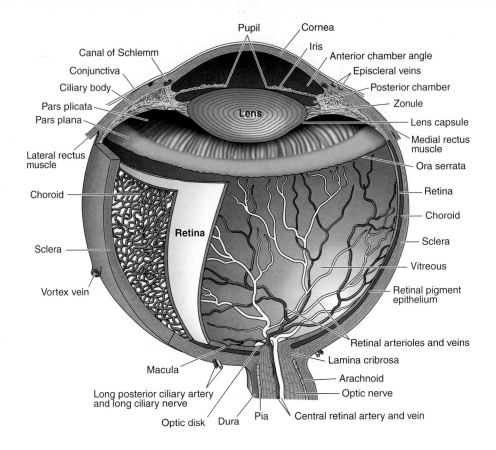

Figure 1-1 *Internal structures of the human eye.* (Redrawn from an original drawing by Paul Peck from: *The Anatomy of the Eye.* Courtesy of Lederle Laboratories. Used by permission from Vaughan D, Asbury T, Riordan-Eva P. *General Ophthalmology,* 15th ed. Stamford, CT: Appleton & Lange, 1999.)

CHAPTER 1 ANATOMY

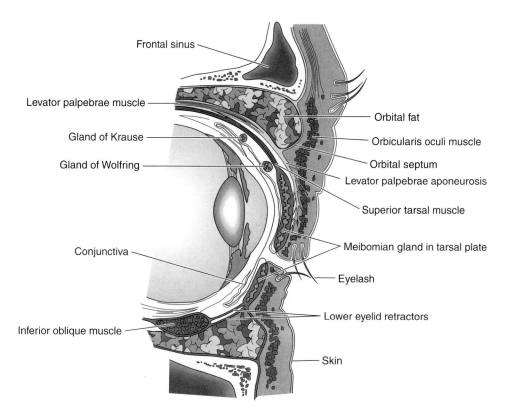

Figure 1-2 *Cross section of the eyelids.*
(Courtesy of C Beard. Used by permission from Vaughan D, Asbury T, Riordan-Eva P. *General Ophthalmology,* 15th ed. Stamford, CT: Appleton & Lange, 1999.)

LACRIMAL APPARATUS The lacrimal apparatus (Fig. 1-3) consists of the lacrimal glands located in the anterior superior temporal segment of the orbit, punctae, canaliculi, lacrimal sac, and nasolacrimal duct, all located in the medial canthus. Tears are produced in the palpebral and orbital portions of the lacrimal gland and secreted onto the conjunctiva via ten secretory ducts. The tears are spread and distributed by capillary action and the blinking motion of the eyelids. Tears drain to the superior and inferior puncta. These two small openings are located on their respective eyelid margin on the lateral border of the medial canthus. Fluid entering the punctae drains through the inferior and superior canaliculi to the common canaliculus, lacrimal sac, and finally, through the nasolacrimal duct into the inferior meatus of the nose.

Tear fluid forms a layer that ranges from 4 to 9 μm thick and serves to protect and lubricate the surface of the cornea, to provide nutrition and oxygenation to the cornea, and to flatten any minor irregularities in the surface of the cornea, providing a uniform optical surface. The tear fluid consists of a lipid layer secreted from the meibomian glands of the eyelids, an aqueous layer produced by the lacrimal apparatus, and a mucous layer produced by the conjunctival goblet cells. Tear fluid has a pH between 7.1 and 8.6 and also contains small quantities of albumin, lysozyme, IgG, IgA, urea, inorganic salts, lactate, and cellular debris.

The blood supply of the lacrimal glands is from a branch of the lacrimal artery and drains into the ophthalmic vein. Lymphatic drainage travels to the preauricular nodes. The lacrimal gland receives sensory innervation from the lacrimal branch of CN V_1, parasympathetic secretory innervation from the superior salivary nucleus via the greater superficial petrosal nerve, and sympathetic innervation from nerve fibers traveling with the lacrimal artery and nerve.

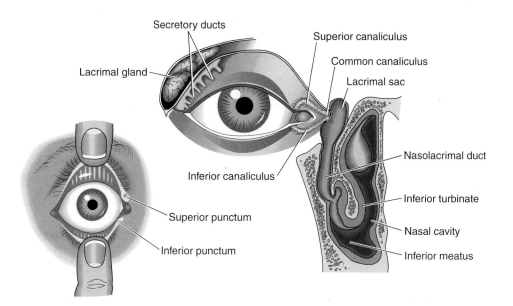

Figure 1-3 *The lacrimal drainage system.*
(Redrawn with modifications from Thompson J, Elstrom ER: Radiography of the nasolacrimal passageways. *Med Radiogr Photogr* 1949;25[3]:66. Used by permission from Vaughan D, Asbury T, Riordan-Eva P. *General Ophthalmology,* 15th ed. Stamford, CT: Appleton & Lange, 1999.)

ANTERIOR SEGMENT

CONJUNCTIVA   The conjunctiva is a thin mucous membrane that covers the posterior surface of the eyelids and the anterior surface of the eyeball itself. The palpebral conjunctiva begins at the eyelid margins and covers the entire surface of the inner eyelid to the fornix, where it is firmly attached to the underlying fibrous tissue, before being reflected back to cover the globe as the bulbar conjunctiva. At the point at which the conjunctiva is reflected back over sclera, the conjunctiva has numerous folds that allow the eye to move freely.

CORNEA   The cornea is a thin, clear, avascular structure that makes up the anterior wall of the globe and functions to refract light toward the pupil and lens. The transition from the cornea to the sclera is the limbus and contains the epithelial stem cells that are the source of the corneal epithelium. The cornea is normally completely avascular. The cornea derives its nourishment from the diffusion of nutrients from the tear fluid anteriorly and aqueous humor posteriorly. Additionally, the superficial layers of the cornea can obtain oxygen from the atmosphere by direct diffusion. The cornea is richly innervated from branches of CN V_1 and even the smallest abrasion results in significant pain.

The cornea itself is divided into five layers (Fig. 1-4): the epithelium, Bowman's layer, the stroma, Descemet's membrane, and the endothelium. The epithelium is a stratified squamous cell layer that is approximately five cells thick and continuous with the conjunctiva. The epithelium is rapidly proliferating, with actively mitotic cells located at the limbus. Full turnover of the epithelium occurs every seven days. Adjacent to the basement membrane of the epithelium is Bowman's layer, which primarily consists of a layer of compacted collagen fibrils. Underneath Bowman's layer is the stroma, composed of parallel lamellae of collagen fibers held together by a mucopolysaccharide matrix. The stroma forms the bulk of the cornea. Descemet's membrane, located beneath the stroma, is tightly associated with the underlying endothelium. The endothelium is one cell thick and lacks any substantial proliferative capacity. The endothelium functions to remove fluid from the stroma to help maintain corneal clarity.

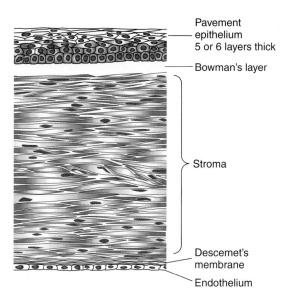

Pavement epithelium
5 or 6 layers thick

Bowman's layer

Stroma

Descemet's membrane

Endothelium

Figure 1-4 *Transverse section of cornea.* (From Wolff E: *Anatomy of the Eye and Orbit,* 4th ed. Blakiston-McGraw, 1954. Used by permission from Vaughan D, Asbury T, Riordan-Eva P. *General Ophthalmology,* 15th ed. Stamford, CT: Appleton & Lange, 1999.)

ANTERIOR CHAMBER The anterior chamber is a semispherical space bounded anteriorly and laterally by the cornea and posteriorly by the iris (Fig. 1-5). The anterior chamber is optically clear and is filled with aqueous humor. Aqueous humor is a cell-free, low-protein, electrolyte-rich fluid produced by ultrafiltration of the serum by the ciliary body. The aqueous flows from the ciliary body through the pupillary opening toward the periphery, where it is filtered through a trabecular meshwork and drained via the canal of Schlem into the scleral sinus and anterior ciliary veins.

IRIS AND LENS The iris is a thickened flat disk of tissue containing a central opening, the pupil (see Fig. 1-5). As the anterior extension of the ciliary body, the iris serves as the dividing mark between the anterior and posterior chambers. It is surrounded both anteriorly and posteriorly by aqueous and sits directly in front of the lens. Within the iris lie the sphincter and dilator muscles of the pupil that serve to adjust the amount of light reaching the retina. The posterior surface of the iris is lined with a double layer of thickened, pigmented epithelial cells. The density of the iris stroma just anterior to this layer is responsible for eye color. The circumferential margin of the iris is attached to the ciliary body.

Directly behind the iris is the lens, which is an avascular, biconvex disk approximately 4 mm thick and 9 mm in diameter. It contains no nerve fibers or lymphatics. The lens focuses the incoming light from the pupil onto the retina. Radiating from the equatorial plane of the lens are zonular fibers that connect to muscles in the ciliary body. Alteration of the tension of the fibers through ciliary muscle contraction and relaxation changes the shape of the lens. This allows for accommodation and the focusing on both near and far objects.

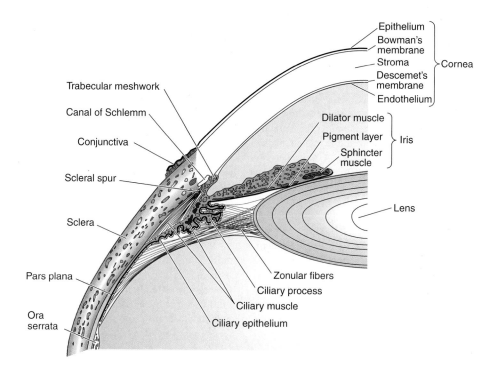

Figure 1-5 *Anterior chamber angle and surrounding structures.* (Used by permission from Vaughan D, Asbury T, Riordan-Eva P. *General Ophthalmology,* 15th ed. Stamford, CT: Appleton & Lange, 1999.)

POSTERIOR SEGMENT
(SEE FIG. 1-1)

VITREOUS   The vitreous makes up almost two thirds of the volume of the eye and is responsible for maintaining the shape of the eyeball. It is a thick, gelatinous fluid surrounded by a hyaloid membrane. The vitreous is located behind the lens and is related anteriorly to the posterior capsule of the lens and posteriorly to the retina. The vitreous is optically clear, but may have suspended fibrous strands and debris.

RETINA   The retina (Fig. 1-6) forms the innermost membrane of the posterior segment of the eye. The optic nerve and retinal vessels enter the retina at the optic disk, a yellow depressed circle. Lateral and slightly inferior to the optic disk is the macula. In the center of the macula is the fovea, which contains the highest density of photoreceptors, permitting the greatest visual acuity. The visual field is centered at the fovea.

The retina is neural tissue, the axons of which travel within the optic nerve. It consists of two layers: the inner neurosensory layer and the outer retinal pigment epithelium layer. The neurosensory layer contains the photoreceptor cells and relay circuits for transmitting light received by the photoreceptors to the brain. The retinal pigment epithelium layer consists of epithelial cells that help to support the metabolic and sensory functions of the neurosensory cell layer.

Vascular supply to the anterior layers of the retina comes from the central retinal artery and its branches, which can be easily visualized on funduscopic examination. The posterior one third of the retina is nourished via diffusion of nutrients from the choroid.

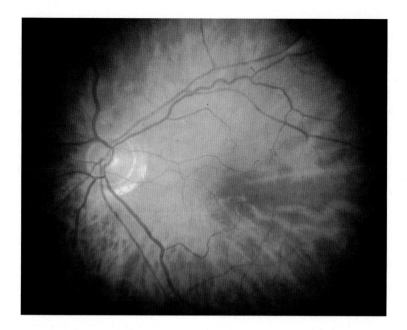

Figure 1-6 *Normal left retina. The yellowish optic nerve has arteries and veins radiating outward from it. The darker pigmented area to the right of the optic nerve is the fovea.*

CHOROID Deep to the retina is the choroid, which provides nutrients to the posterior layers of the retina. The choroid is the most posterior portion of the uveal tract, which also includes the ciliary body and the iris. It is a highly vascularized connective tissue layer located between the retina and sclera.

SCLERA The sclera is a thick white fibrous layer that forms the outer posterior wall of the eye, deep to the choroid. It is connected circumferentially to the cornea anteriorly and merges within the dura of the optic nerve posteriorly. Approximately 1 mm thick, it is nourished by vessels coursing through the episclera, its outer elastic covering. The sclera provides structural integrity to the eye as well as attachment for the extraocular muscles.

EXTRAOCULAR MUSCLES The eye has six cardinal directions of movement and is controlled by six extraocular muscles (EOM) (Table 1-1). The EOM are innervated by CN III, IV, and VI. The superior and inferior recti muscles are the primary controls for vertical eye movement. The medial and lateral recti move the eye in the horizontal plane. The recti muscles are attached to the sclera 5 to 8-mm posterior to the limbus and to a tendinous band in the posterior orbit known as the annulus of Zinn.

The superior oblique muscle originates on the orbital wall near the superior medial border of the annulus, stretches around the pulley-like trochlea located on the superior medial portion of the orbit. The superior oblique moves the eye inward and downward. The inferior oblique is the only muscle not attached near the optic canal. Rather, it runs from the anterior medial portion of the orbit to the posterior lateral portion of the sclera. Contraction of the inferior oblique causes outward and upward eye movement.

ORBIT The eye sits in the orbital cavity that is formed by bones of the cranium and the face. These bones serve to protect the eye while allowing it to move freely in multiple directions. The following bones contribute to the orbit (Fig. 1-7): maxilla, frontal, sphenoid, zygomatic, palatine, ethmoid, and lacrimal. The medial and inferior walls of the orbit are the thinnest and are most commonly fractured with trauma to the eye and orbit. Surrounding the globe is loose fatty tissue cushioning the eye against injuries and allowing free movement of the eye.

The orbit contains multiple fossae for accommodating such structures as the lacrimal apparatus, lacrimal sac, and trochlea and foramina which allow the transmission of nerves and veins to the eye (Table 1-2).

TABLE 1-1 FEATURES OF THE EXTRAOCULAR MUSCLES

Muscle	Innervation	Primary Direction of Eye Movement with Muscle Contraction
Superior rectus	CN III	Elevation
Inferior rectus	CN III	Depression
Medial rectus	CN III	Adduction
Lateral rectus	CN VI	Abduction
Superior oblique	CN IV	Intorsion
Inferior oblique	CN III	Extorsion

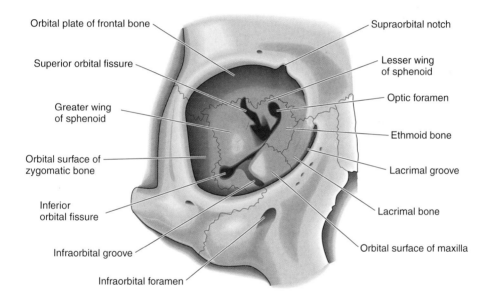

Figure 1-7 *Anterior view of bones of right orbit.* (Used by permission from Vaughan D, Asbury T, Riordan-Eva P. *General Ophthalmology,* 15th ed. Stamford, CT: Appleton & Lange, 1999.)

TABLE 1-2 ORBITAL FOSSAE AND THEIR CONTENTS

Fossa	Bony Location	Contents
Optic canal	Sphenoid bone	Optic nerve Ophthalmic artery and vein
Superior orbital fissure	Greater and lesser wing of sphenoid bone	Lacrimal, frontal, trochlear, oculomotor, abducens, nasociliary nerves Sympathetic root of the ciliary ganglion Superior and inferior orbital veins Recurrent lacrimal artery
Inferior orbital fissure	Greater wing of sphenoid bone and maxillary bone	Infraorbital, zygomatic, pterygopalatine nerves

Chapter 2

BASIC EYE EXAMINATION

SUDHIR R. VORA
SCOTT M. DAMRAUER

CHECKING VISION

The first step in the ophthalmic screening examination involves assessing the status of a patient's visual acuity (Table 2-1.) The examiner assesses vision by using either a standardized visual acuity chart or a near card specially designed for bedside use. If such tools are unavailable, the clinician can attempt to improvise by using such items as a newspaper or food label.

SNELLEN TEST

Although many tests have been devised for assessing a patient's vision, the Snellen test serves as the standard examining method. The Snellen chart (Fig. 2-1) displays lines of numbers and block letters, with the size of the characters decreasing from top to bottom.

To perform the Snellen test:

- Position the patient at a distance of 20 feet (or 14 inches for the near card) away from the chart. Whenever possible, visual acuity should be assessed while the patient is wearing the appropriate glasses or corrective lenses. Patients over 40 years old may require reading glasses or bifocals to overcome age-associated presbyopia when using the reading card.
- Testing each eye separately, ask the patient to read progressively smaller lines on the chart and determine the smallest line that he or she can read with greater than 50 percent accuracy.
- Document the corresponding vision (e.g., 20/20, 20/200) for each eye. The numerator of this fraction represents the distance of the patient from the chart. The denominator represents the distance from which a person with normal visual acuity would read the line with greater than 50 percent accuracy. The abbreviation OD (oculus dexter) represents the right eye and OS (oculus sinister) represents the left eye.

TABLE 2-1   **VISUAL ACUITY**

Acuity	Comments
20/15	Excellent vision
20/20	Normal visual acuity
20/40	Acceptable vision for driving
⋮	⋮
20/200	Legally blind
20/400	Can only see the big E on Snellen letter chart
Counting fingers (CF)	—
Hand motion (HM)	—
Light perception (LP)	—
No light perception (NLP)	Worst

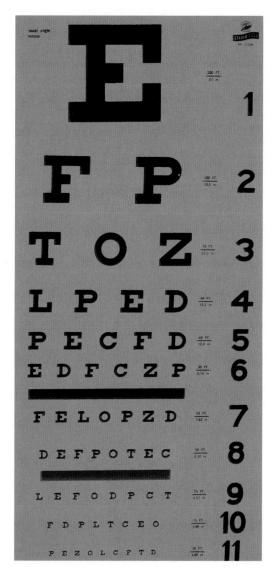

Figure 2-1 *Standard Snellen letter chart. When the patient is 20 feet from the chart, the big E is at the top corresponds to 20/400 vision, and smaller letters toward the bottom are the 20/20 and 20/15 letters.*

NEAR VISION TEST

When performance of the standard Snellen test is impractical, the ER physician can elect to use the near vision test (Fig. 2-2) to assess visual acuity. This test is similar to the standard Snellen test, with the physician placing the near vision card roughly 14 in. from the eyes of the patients and repeating the steps described previously. Although this test is less precise than the Snellen test, it is often sufficient for a gross assessment of acuity.

If the patient has bifocals or reading glasses, the patient should wear these for the exam.

LOW VISION TESTING

For patients with less than 20/400 vision, the examiner may be unable to use the tests described above and should improvise by testing more basic visual functions. In these situations, the clinician may elect to test visual acuity via the more primitive tests described as follows.

COUNTING FINGERS In this test, the clinician determines the distance at which the patient is capable of accurately determining the number of fingers being held up by the examiner. For instance, if the patient is able to count the number of fingers being held up by the clinician from a distance of 3 feet, the results of this test can be recorded as "CF 3 feet" (counting fingers at 3 feet).

HAND MOTION If the patient is unable to count fingers from very short distances, the clinician should attempt to determine whether or not the patient can distinguish vertical hand movements from horizontal hand movements when they are performed by the examiner. If the patient is able to perform this function, the clinician can record this as "HM" (hand motions).

LIGHT PERCEPTION Finally, if the patient's vision is diminished to the point that he or she cannot appreciate hand movements, the examiner can test for light perception by shining a bright light directly onto the patient's eyes and asking whether or not the patient can appreciate the stimulus. Ask the patient to tell you when the light goes on as you move the light back and forth across the eye. Be sure to adequately cover the opposing eye so that no light can be seen. A positive response is recorded as "LP" (light perception) and a negative response is recorded as "NLP" (no light perception).

PIN HOLE ACUITY

If the clinician is attempting to distinguish visual defects resulting from refractive errors (myopia, hyperopia, astigmatism) from pathologic conditions, such as cataracts, optic nerve disease, and so forth, he or she may elect to reevaluate the patient's vision using a pinhole aperture. Such an aperture can be made by punching a hole in a piece of paper with the tip of a pencil. Pinhole testing generally eliminates mild uncorrected refractive errors and so defects in vision detected in pinhole testing can be assumed to result from nonrefractive errors of the eye.

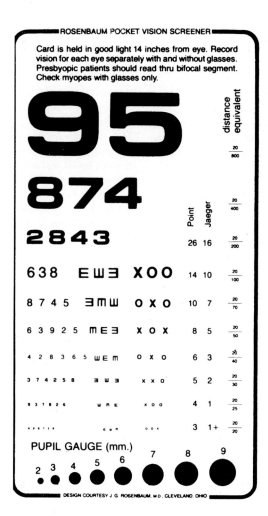

Figure 2-2 *The near card is for measuring reading acuity and is held at 14 ins. Patients should wear any prescribed glasses or bifocals when reading the smaller print.*

VISUAL FIELDS TESTING

Defects in visual field testing (Figs. 2-3 and 2-4) can indicate injury at any point along the visual pathway leading from the retina to the occipital lobe. Goldmann and Humphrey visual fields are more formal methods for measuring visual fields, but confrontational fields provide a gross assessment of the periphery.

CONFRONTATIONAL VISUAL FIELDS

To perform a confrontational visual field:

- Place yourself in front of the patient at arm's length.
- Ask the patient to cover one eye and to fixate on your nose with the open eye.
- Ask the patient to report when he or she first sees your fingers as you move your hands into the field of view from various regions in the periphery. In this manner, map out the patient's visual field and take special note of regions in space that the patient is unable to visually appreciate.
- Next, with one hand in each of the superior quadrants, simultaneously display fingers on both hands and ask the patient to determine the total number of fingers that are being displayed. Repeat for the inferior quadrants. If the patient is unable to count the total number of fingers displayed simultaneously on both hands, record this as an abnormality, since it may indicate a neglect syndrome.
- Finally, repeat the steps for the patient's other eye.

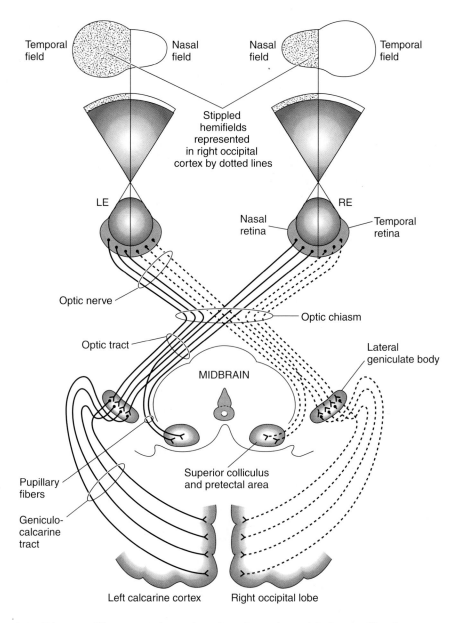

Figure 2-3 *Diagram of the nerve pathways from the retina to the occipital cortex. Visual information is topographically organized, and this relationship is maintained throughout the system.*

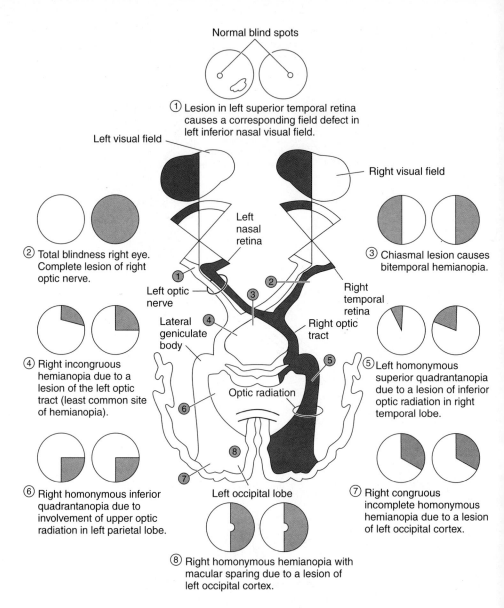

Normal blind spots

① Lesion in left superior temporal retina causes a corresponding field defect in left inferior nasal visual field.

Left visual field

Right visual field

Left nasal retina

② Total blindness right eye. Complete lesion of right optic nerve.

③ Chiasmal lesion causes bitemporal hemianopia.

Left optic nerve

Right temporal retina

Right optic tract

Lateral geniculate body

④ Right incongruous hemianopia due to a lesion of the left optic tract (least common site of hemianopia).

⑤ Left homonymous superior quadrantanopia due to a lesion of inferior optic radiation in right temporal lobe.

Optic radiation

⑥ Right homonymous inferior quadrantanopia due to involvement of upper optic radiation in left parietal lobe.

Left occipital lobe

⑦ Right congruous incomplete homonymous hemianopia due to a lesion of left occipital cortex.

⑧ Right homonymous hemianopia with macular sparing due to a lesion of left occipital cortex.

Figure 2-4 *Lesions of the optic pathway and corresponding visual field defects.*

PUPILLARY EXAMINATION

The pupillary examination is intended to allow the clinician to detect functional deficits in the pupillary reflex arc, the neural circuitry that allows the eye to respond to light via pupillary constriction. Since there is equal bilateral innervation of the pupils, both pupils normally respond in an identical fashion to a light stimulus directed at either eye. The entire examination is summarized in the following steps.

- Ask the patient to fixate on a distant object in a darkened room.
- Shine a penlight onto the patient's face being careful not to place the light beam directly onto either pupil.
- Measure the pupillary diameter in both eyes with a small ruler. Take note of both the absolute size of each pupil and also the relation between the two.
- Next, shine the penlight directly onto the pupil of one eye. Gauge the degree of pupillary constriction as well as the rapidity of the response. Also note the degree of constriction and rapidity of response for the other eye (consensual reflex). Perform this test for both eyes and record the results. Absence of the pupillary constriction response in a given eye can signal either an afferent or efferent neuronal defect, but the two can be distinguished by the swinging light test (Fig. 2-5).
- To perform the swinging light test, swing a penlight back and forth between the two pupils. When the light focuses on one eye, its pupil should constrict with consensual constriction of the opposite pupil. When the light reaches the opposite eye, this pupil should now constrict with consensual constriction in the other eye. In the case of an afferent defect, such as optic nerve damage, an eye will be able to constrict consensually but will dilate when the beam of light is swung directly onto it from the opposite side. This is known as a Marcus-Gunn pupil (Fig. 2-6).
- Finally, test for accommodation by asking the patient to fixate on your finger at a distance of 1 foot. The ability to accommodate is intact if pupillary constriction is evident as you move your finger closer and closer to the patient.

Light stimulus on the right eye

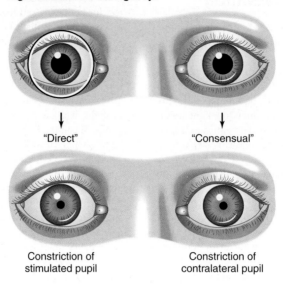

"Direct"   "Consensual"

Constriction of   Constriction of
stimulated pupil   contralateral pupil

Figure 2-5   *When a light is shone into one eye, both the right and left pupils will constrict equally in a normal patient.*

Diffuse illumination

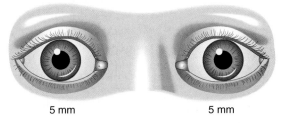

5 mm   5 mm

Light on normal left eye

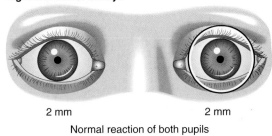

2 mm   2 mm

Normal reaction of both pupils

Light on eye with afferent defect

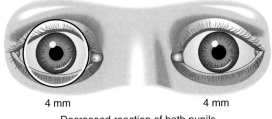

4 mm   4 mm

Decreased reaction of both pupils

Figure 2-6 *Normal constriction of both pupils occurs when the light is shone into the normal left eye. When the light is moved to the right eye, the pupils are less constricted, representing an afferent pupillary defect of the right eye.*

MOTILITY EXAMINATION

Movement in each eye is controlled by six extraocular muscles (superior, inferior, medial, and lateral recti and superior and inferior obliques). The function and innervation of these muscles is described in Table 2-2.

The motility examination can be performed as follows.

- Ask the patient to follow your finger with both eyes as you move it in the cardinal fields of gaze.
- With each movement, note whether the amplitude is normal or abnormal. For instance, when the eyes are moving from right to left or from left to right, the nasal sclera of the adducting eye should disappear completely with maximum displacement. When the eyes are moving up, half of the cornea should disappear behind the upper eyelid. Finally, when the eyes are moving down, two thirds of the cornea should disappear behind the lower eyelid.
- If bilateral eye movements are abnormal, perform the test in each eye separately with the other eye covered.
- Record any sign of nystagmus and the ocular movements that give rise to it.

TABLE 2-2   **ACTION AND INNERVATION OF THE EXTRAOCULAR MUSCLES**

Extraocular Muscle	Function	Innervation
Lateral rectus	Abduction	CN VI
Superior oblique	Abduction, depression, and intortion	CN IV
Medial rectus	Adduction	CN III
Inferior rectus	Depression	CN III
Superior rectus	Elevation	CN III
Inferior oblique	Abduction, elevation, and intortion	CN III

EXTERNAL EXAMINATION

External examination entails a careful inspection of both the ocular surface of the eye and surrounding structures. The examiner must inspect the eye thoroughly, everting both the upper and lower eyelids to obtain a clear view of both the cornea and conjunctiva (Fig. 2-7). The examiner should also ask the patient to shift gaze direction to provide a more complete view of eye structures. For a more careful analysis of the eye surface, the examiner may elect to perform corneal staining. In the procedure, the clinician first anesthetizes the eye with topical anesthetic and then places a wet fluorescein strip in the conjunctival cul-de-sac of the eye. Green patches on the corneal surface of the eye that do not go away on blinking can be corneal abrasions or defects. Use of a cobalt blue light (or Wood's lamp) will cause areas of fluorescein staining to glow green.

Careful consideration should be given not only to the examination of the globe, but also to its positioning within the eye socket. For instance, exopthalmos (protrusion of the eyeball) can signal underlying Graves' disease, orbital inflammation, or an orbital tumor. Finally, the clinician should note the appearance and position of the eyelid (Fig. 2-8). Ptosis of the eye could result from CN III palsy, Horner's syndrome, or myasthenia gravis.

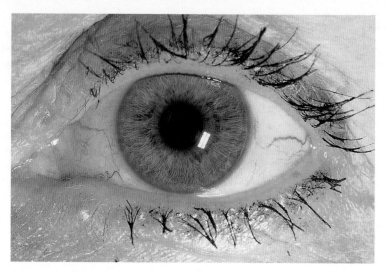

Figure 2-7 *Appearance of the normal eye. Note the shiny light reflex from the cornea, indicative of a smooth corneal surface. Mascara can be seen on the eyelashes and eyelid margin.*

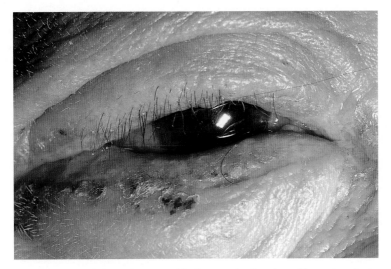

Figure 2-8 *Eyelid vesicles caused by herpes simplex virus. The patient had concomitant herpetic corneal disease.*

SLIT LAMP EXAMINATION

Examination via a slit lamp biomicroscope allows for an accurate and magnified look at the anatomy of the anterior chamber of the eye. The patient places the chin on the chin rest attached to the biomicroscope and the forehead forward against the forehead rest. The clinician sets the oculars initially at zero and adjusts the width to his or her interpupillary distance. Focusing is controlled by moving the chassis itself for course adjustments or by moving the joystick backward and forward for fine adjustment. Finally, the clinician can control the shape of the light beam itself, which varies from a broad band to a tiny slit (Fig. 2-9A). Specific methods of mechanical adjustment depend on the particular model and design of the biomicroscope.

Using this apparatus, the clinician can examine the eyelids, conjunctiva, cornea, anterior chamber, iris, lens, and the vitreous of each eye (Fig. 2-9B).

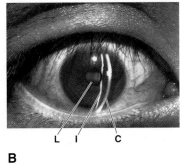

B

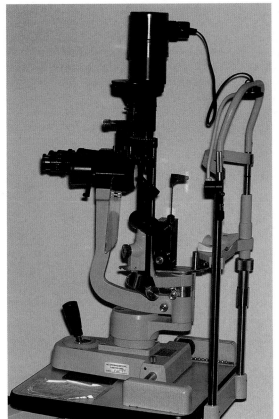

A

Figure 2-9 *A. The slit lamp biomicroscope provides a magnified view of the eye. This particular model is known as the Haag-Streit 900. B. A thin slit permits the differentiation and examination of ocular structures. C = cornea, I = iris, L = lens.*

INTRAOCULAR PRESSURE

Normal values for intraocular pressure (IOP) range from 8 to 21 mm Hg. Abnormal values can range from as low as 0 mm Hg, in cases such as that of a ruptured globe, to 40 mm Hg or higher, observed in certain types of glaucoma. There are many different techniques for measuring intraocular pressure, the most common of which are described as follows.

APPLANATION TONOMETRY

The applanation tonometer is an easy to use and accurate device that is usually found on most slit lamps (Fig. 2-10). Alternatively, a hand-held applanation device is available to be used with patients who are unable to position themselves properly in front of the slit lamp biomicroscope. The examiner begins by first anesthetizing the eye to be tested and adding a drop of fluoroscein dye. The applanation tonometer measures the force required to flatten the anterior surface of the eye by a fixed amount. The higher the intraocular pressure, the greater the amount of force that is required to flatten the eye and the higher the pressure reading. The dial on the tonometer is turned until the inner edges of the semicircles touch (Fig. 2-11). This method serves as the gold standard for measuring intraocular pressure.

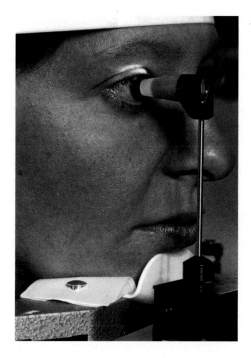

Figure 2-10 *Applanation tonometry using the Goldmann tonometer. Anesthetic drops are instilled into the eye and the tonometer lightly compresses the anterior cornea.*

Dial reading greater than pressure of globe

Dial reading less than pressure of globe

Dial reading equals pressure of globe

Figure 2-11 *When the inside edges of the semicircles touch, the intraocular pressure can be read from the dial.*

SCHIOTZ TONOMETRY

This device, although somewhat less accurate than the applanation tonometer, is more broadly available in most clinical settings (Fig. 2-12 and 2-13). The instrument works by applying a fixed weight to the eyeball while the patient is in supine position and then measuring the resulting degree of indentation. Increased intraocular pressure results in greater resistance to indentation, such that there is an inverse relationship between the degree of indentation and the pressure within the eye. The tonometer consists of a plunger that functions to measure the degree of indentation of the cornea. This value can be converted to an intraocular pressure reading (mm Hg) by a conversion table that is provided with the instrument. The major disadvantages of this technique include risk of infection or trauma to the eye with use.

MANUAL ASSESSMENT

Manual assessment provides a crude measurement of intraocular pressure but one that may be useful in the absence of a tonometer. The patient is asked to close both eyes and the examiner then uses the index and middle finger of each hand to palpate the globe through the upper eyelid. By palpating in this fashion, the clinician can detect any gross differences in pressure between the two eyes. The eye with greater pressure will feel firmer on palpation than the unaffected eye. This method should be avoided in eyes that have undergone recent surgery or if there is suspected rupture of the globe.

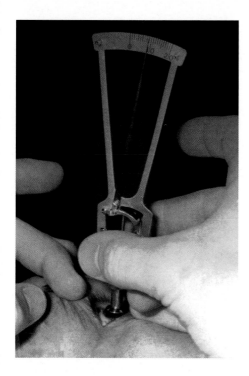

Figure 2-12 *Schiotz tonometry measurement on a supine patient. The displacement of the needle on the Schiotz tonometer can be converted into a pressure reading.*

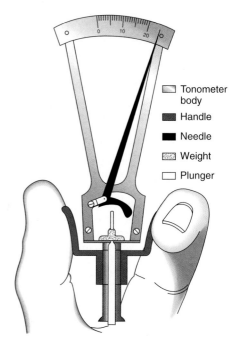

Tonometer body

Handle

Needle

Weight

Plunger

Figure 2-13 *Diagram of the Schiotz tonometer. The tonometer is held as shown so that no external pressure is applied to the eye.*

FUNDUSCOPY

DIRECT FUNDUSCOPIC EXAMINATION

Direct examination of the fundus of the eye via ophthalmoscopy (Fig. 2-14) provides the physician with a direct and magnified view at the posterior segment of the eye. This procedure is particularly useful in diagnosing diseases of the retina such as diabetic retinopathy and retinal occlusion and for optic nerve pathology such as papilledema and glaucoma. The ophthalmoscope is an instrument with multiple apertures, thereby allowing the clinician to adjust for varying pupil size from one patient to another. This instrument also has an illumination source, a set of objective lenses that allow for focusing, and filters that provide enhanced contrast. For instance, the green filter found on most ophthalmoscopes serves to enhance visualization of the retinal nerve fiber layer, retinal blood vessels, and retinal hemorrhages by increasing their contrast with the surrounding retinal tissue. The following is the procedure for direct funduscopy. If available, instill dilating drops (phenylephrine 2.5%, tropicamide 1%). The dilated pupil will permit an easier view of the retina and more thorough peripheral retinal examination.

- Hold the ophthalmoscope in the right hand for visualization of the right eye and in the left hand for visualization of the left eye. Visualize the right eye with your right eye and the left eye of the patient with your left eye.

- Have the patient fixate straight ahead or slightly to the temporal side.
- Set the ophthalmoscope to 7 to 10 diopters and focus light onto the patient's pupil from a slight temporal angle at a distance of 4 to 6 in., until the red reflex is visualized. Absence of a red reflex could result from corneal or lens opacities or blood in the vitreous.
- While slowly moving toward the eye with the ophthalmoscope, dial back the diopteric power of the ophthalmoscope until the retina is visualized.
- Once the retina is visualized, follow the major vascular channels in the retina as they converge onto the head of the optic nerve (Fig. 2-15).
- Carefully observe the optic nerve, looking for such things as pallor, a large cup to disk ratio, neovascularization, or the lack of a sharp edge between the optic disk and the surrounding retina (Fig. 2-16).
- Look at the vessels of the fundus for evidence of focal narrowing, arteriovenous thickening, emboli, and attenuation.
- Next, look temporally from the optic disk to visualize the macula and fovea of the eye, looking for evidence of macular degeneration or diabetes.
- Finally, scan the retina for signs of pathology, such as tears, pigment clumping, or hemorrhage. The various pathologies evident upon funduscopic examination are detailed in the chapters that follow.

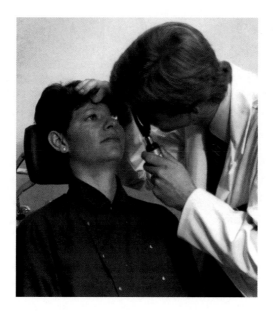

Figure 2-14 *Direct ophthalmoscopy provides a view of the retina and optic nerve. The examiner's eye, the opening on the ophthalmoscope, and the patient's pupil must be coaxial.*

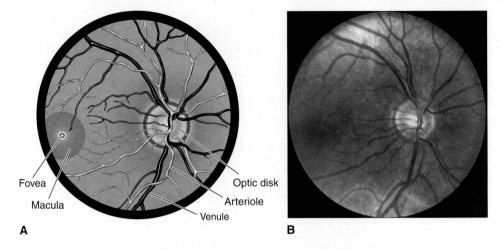

Figure 2-15 *A. Diagram of the posterior portion of the retina and optic nerve. The location of the optic nerve can be found by following the blood vessels. **B.** Corresponding retinal fundus photograph.*

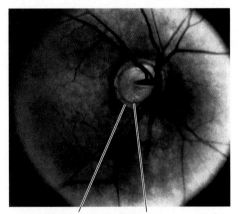

Edge of disk   Edge of cup

Figure 2-16 *The cup is a depression (and slight color change) in the center of the optic nerve. The ratio of the diameter of the cup to the disk is important in conditions such as glaucoma.*

INDIRECT OPHTHALMOSCOPY (SEE FIGURE 2-17)

Indirect ophthalmoscopy allows the physician to examine the posterior pole and retinal periphery. With the use of a 20 or 28 diopter handheld lens and a specialized headset which contains a light source, prisms, and converging lenses, the oph-thalmologist has a wide-angle view of the retina with less magnification than with the direct oph-thalmoscope. Retinal hemorrhages, scars, and other pathology stand out against the normal background retina. With scleral indentation, the far periphery of the retina can be visualized. Retinal tears and breaks in this region are often located in this area.

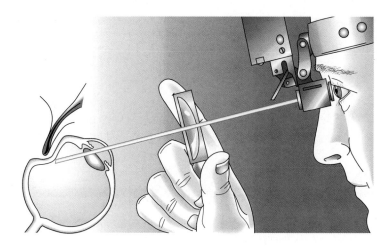

Figure 2-17   *Indirect ophthalmoscopy uses a specialized headset and lenses to view the posterior pole. This provides a wider field of view, but with less magnification than the direct ophthalmoscope. Indentation of the sclera permits viewing of the most peripheral retina.*

COLOR VISION TESTING

Color vision testing is used primarily to detect abnormalities in the retina (congenital red–green color blindness, rod–cone photoreceptor dystrophies, etc.) or the optic nerve (optic neuritis, compressive optic neuropathy, etc.). Standardized color plates (Ishihara, HRR-

AO) contain colored dots of colors commonly confused (Fig. 2-18). Patients with color vision deficits are unable to read the numbers on these plates. The first plate of each series is the control plate—even patients with color vision deficits should be able to see these numbers. Other more formal color vision tests include the Farnsworth D-15 and 100 hue tests.

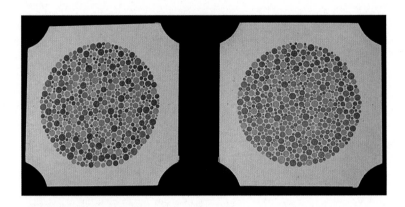

Figure 2-18 *The numbers on the color plates are a hue that can be easily confused with the background in color-deficient patients.*

STEREOACUITY TESTING

Stereoacuity is a measurement of how well the two eyes function together for depth perception and discernment of three-dimensional objects. The patient wears polarized glasses (Fig. 2-19).

The stereo plates are also polarized so that each eye sees a slightly disparate image. The brain combines the two images to create a three-dimensional image. Patients who suppress the vision in one eye will not be able to discern any three-dimensional effect.

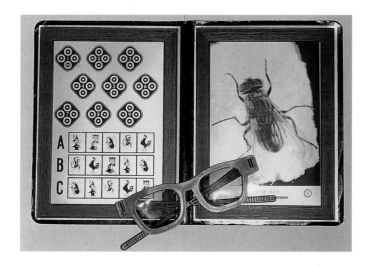

Figure 2-19 *Stereoacuity testing using polarized plates and glasses.*

Chapter 3

TRAUMA

LAUREN SHATZ

CORINA STANCEY

CORNEAL FOREIGN BODY

HISTORY

- Activity at time of injury (grinding, sanding, or hammering objects)
- Material involved (metal, glass, wood, dirt, cement)
- Attempts to remove or wash out foreign body
- Use of protective eyewear

FINDINGS ON EXAMINATION

COMMON

- Foreign body on surface of cornea (Fig. 3-1)
- Epithelial disruption around foreign body
- Corneal infiltrate (Fig. 3-2)
- Rust rings occurring with iron-containing foreign bodies
- Lid swelling
- Conjunctival injection
- Conjunctival foreign bodies
- Tearing
- Blepharospasm
- Linear streaks on epithelium (suggestive of foreign material embedded under lid)

LESS COMMON

- Corneal laceration
- Cell and flare
- Hyphema
- Hypopyon—suggestive of infection

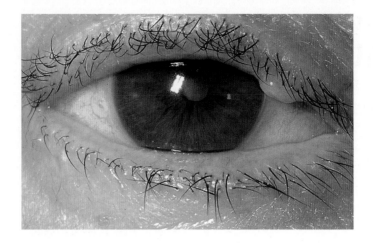

Figure 3-1   *Small fleck of metallic debris on the cornea nasal to the pupil.*

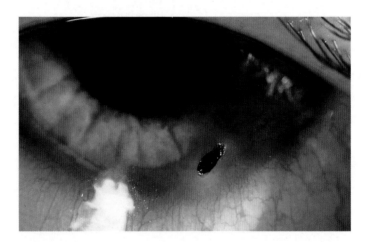

Figure 3-2   *Corneal infiltrate and dilated limbal blood vessels in this patient with a foreign body that has been present for several days.*

EXAMINATION OUTLINE

If the injury is from cement, plaster, or other chemical, immediately irrigate the eye and defer examination (see section "Chemical and Thermal Injury")

- Instill topical anesthetic if patient is uncomfortable
- Check visual acuity
- Check pupils
- Slit lamp examination with instillation of fluorescein to assess epithelial defects
- Perform Seidel test if suspicion of penetrating ocular injury exists
- Evert upper lid to look for debris (if a ruptured globe is suspected, avoid lid eversion as this maneuver may apply pressure on the globe)
- Sweep conjunctival fornices with moistened cotton swab
- Dilated fundus exam, x-ray, CT scan, and MRI may be indicated if intraocular or intraorbital foreign body is suspected (MRI is contraindicated in cases of suspected metallic foreign body)

TREATMENT

- Superficial foreign bodies may be removed with irrigation or a moistened cotton swab
- Shallowly embedded foreign bodies may be dislodged with the tip of a 25-gauge needle while at the slit lamp
- Once foreign body is removed, treat with broad-spectrum antibiotic drops or ointment; a cycloplegic agent (cyclopentolate 1% QID or scopolamine 0.25% TID) may improve ocular comfort if patient is photophobic

FOLLOW UP

Refer urgently if:

- Any corneal laceration
- Positive Seidel test (leakage of intraocular fluid present)

- Evidence of corneal ulcer or infiltrate
- Deeply embedded foreign body
- Hypopyon or significant anterior chamber reaction
- After treatment of uncomplicated corneal foreign body, follow up with ophthalmologist in 24 to 48 hours is recommended.

PEARLS

- Industrial injuries involving plaster, cement, mortar, and whitewash may also cause an alkali injury as these substances contain lime. Irrigate thoroughly and check pH. Persistently elevated tear pH suggests retained foreign material in the upper or lower fornices (see section "Chemical and Thermal Injury").

- Metallic foreign bodies, although often sterile, can cause a significant inflammatory response in the corneal stroma and epithelium due to rust and chemicals on the foreign body.

- Glass, sand, and ceramic materials are frequently inert and can be left in place if the surface epithelium has healed over and there is no significant inflammatory reaction.

- Wood and other organic foreign bodies can harbor bacteria or fungi and are highly inflammatory.

ICD-9 CODES

374.8	Retained foreign body of eyelid
930.0	Corneal foreign body
930.1	Foreign body conjunctival sac

CPT CODES

65205	Removal of conjunctival foreign body
65222	Removal of corneal foreign body

CORNEAL ABRASION

HISTORY

- Description of event causing injury, usually blunt trauma
- Discomfort ranging from foreign body sensation to sharp pain worse with blinking
- History of recurrent corneal "erosion" syndrome (see Recurrent Erosion Syndrome)

FINDINGS ON EXAMINATION

- Pain relieved by topical anesthetic
- Copious, watery tearing
- Photophobia
- Blepharospasm and lid swelling
- Irregular epithelium or area of missing epithelium (Fig. 3-3)
- Fluorescein staining on cornea highlighting an epithelial defect (Fig. 3-4)
- Absence of corneal infiltrate
- Negative Seidel test
- Conjunctival injection
- Mild cell and flare

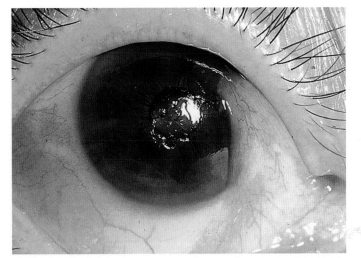

A

B

Figure 3-3 *A. The epithelial edge is irregular in this central corneal abrasion. B. The area of involved epithelium is highlighted by the fluorescein dye.*

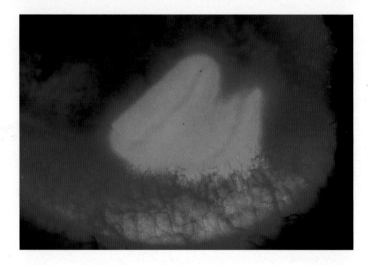

Figure 3-4 *Loose flap of corneal epithelium. When stained with fluorescein dye, the edges of the flap are more prominent. The dye also diffuses under the loose epithelium making the abrasion appear larger than the area of loose epithelium.*

EXAMINATION OUTLINE

- Instill topical anesthetic
- Check visual acuity
- Check pupil reactivity
- Slit lamp examination
- Stain surface of cornea with fluorescein dye
- Lid eversion to locate a foreign body

TREATMENT

- Topical antibiotic ointment or drops QID (erythromycin, polymyxin–bacitracin)
- Contact lens wearers require coverage for gram-negative bacteria, particularly *Pseudomonas* (tobramycin, ofloxacin, or ciprofloxacin)
- Cycloplegic agents reduce discomfort by inhibiting ciliary body spasm (cyclopentolate 1% or 2% QID, scopolamine 0.25% TID)
- Pressure patching at patient's request (avoid patching if suspicion for infection exists)
- Topical NSAID agents are helpful in the short term management of pain (ketorolac 0.5% QID or diclofenac 0.1% QID)

FOLLOW UP

- Patients with large abrasions or abrasions in the visual axis should be examined the next day
- Small and peripheral abrasions may be followed 2 to 5 days after initiating treatment

- Contact lens wearers should be seen daily and may resume contact lens wear once the eye has felt normal for 1 week while off medication

PEARLS

- Topical anesthetics should *never* be prescribed since they inhibit epithelial healing
- Avoid patching contact lens wearers and patients who sustained injury from vegetable matter or a fingernail
- Yellow, purulent discharge is highly suspicious for an infection
- A corneal infiltrate is suggestive of infection and warrants urgent ophthalmologic consultation
- Vertical, linear staining on the cornea is common with a foreign body lodged under the lid
- Traumatic corneal abrasion, particularly with paper edges and fingernails, may lead to recurrent corneal erosion syndrome.

ICD-9 CODE

918.1   Corneal abrasion

RECURRENT EROSION SYNDROME

HISTORY

- Prior corneal abrasion, especially those caused by paper, fingernail, or tree branch.
- Recurrent episodes of acute eye pain or discomfort, tearing, and photophobia caused by sudden detachment of corneal epithelium from an irregular basement membrane.
- Often occurs upon awakening from sleep or after rubbing the eye.

EXAMINATION OUTLINE

- Slit lamp examination of the cornea may reveal areas of irregular corneal epithelium or a focal epithelial defect.
- Loose, poorly adherent sheets of epithelium are present.

TREATMENT

- Treat in a similar fashion to corneal abrasion.
- Further management provided by the ophthalmologist may include more long-term treatments such as hypertonic saline drops, epithelial debridement, bandage soft contact lens, anterior stromal puncture, and phototherapeutic keratectomy.

ICD-9 CODE

371.42   Recurrent erosion of cornea

CONJUNCTIVAL AND CORNEAL LACERATION

HISTORY

- Description of event causing injury, (i.e., often sharp foreign body entering eye)
- If foreign body injury, determine the source, composition, and trajectory of the material and possible intraocular retention of foreign material
- Prior tetanus immunization

FINDINGS ON EXAMINATION

CONJUNCTIVAL LACERATION (FIG. 3-5)

- Hemorrhagic and swollen conjunctival edges
- Exposure of underlying sclera and episclera
- Staining of the edges of the laceration with fluorescein dye

PARTIAL-THICKNESS CORNEAL LACERATION (FIG. 3-6)

- Epithelial defect
- Deep anterior chamber
- Negative Seidel test
- Hyphema or microhyphema
- Normal intraocular pressure

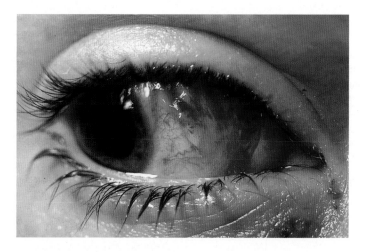

Figure 3-5 *Conjunctival laceration nasal to the limbus. The hemorrhagic and edematous conjunctiva has retracted slightly toward the caruncle. The underlying sclera is visible through the laceration.*

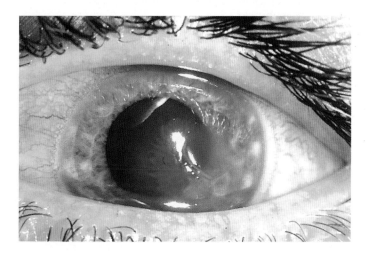

Figure 3-6 *Partial thickness corneal laceration following an injury from a firecracker. The adjacent corneal stroma is hazy from edema. The anterior chamber is intact and well formed.*

**FULL THICKNESS CORNEAL LACERATION
(FIGS. 3-7 AND 3-8)**

- Positive Seidel test
- Irregular pupil with or without iris prolapse
- Shallow anterior chamber
- Hyphema or microhyphema
- Cataract
- Normal or low intraocular pressure (if full thickness laceration is suspected, defer measurement of intraocular pressure)

EXAMINATION OUTLINE

- Check visual acuity—vision may be very poor if laceration involves central cornea
- Assess pupils with penlight
- Slit lamp examination
- Perform Seidel test

TREATMENT

CORNEAL LACERATIONS

- All suspected corneal lacerations require urgent ophthalmologic consultation

- Further examination and treatment may be deferred until the patient receives ophthalmologic care
- Cover the involved eye with a metal shield or the end of a Styrofoam cup; avoid placing pressure on the eye by attaching the tape to the forehead and cheek and instruct the patient not to touch the eye
- Full thickness lacerations frequently require surgical repair
- Partial thickness lacerations are often treated with cycloplegic agents, topical antibiotics, and pressure patching; a bandage soft contact lens or operative repair may be indicated

CONJUNCTIVAL LACERATIONS

- Conjunctival lacerations often heal with antibiotic prophylaxis
- Debride loose and necrotic tissue
- With a conjunctival laceration, have high suspicion for a ruptured globe

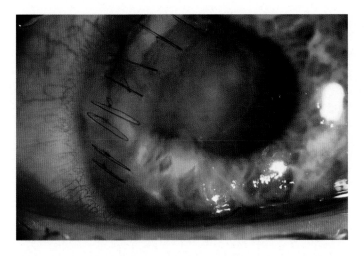

Figure 3-7 *Corneal laceration repaired with nylon sutures. Iris tissue that prolapsed through the wound was unable to be saved and thus left an irregular pupil.*

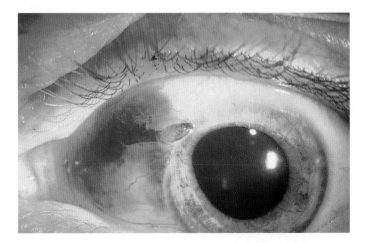

Figure 3-8 *Laceration at corneal limbus with iris prolapse and involvement of adjacent conjunctiva. The pupil is stretched towards the site of the laceration due to the iris prolapse. Subconjunctival hemorrhage surrounds the conjunctival laceration.*

ICD-9 CODES

870.3	Penetrating wound of orbit without mention of foreign body
871.7	Unspecified ocular penetration
871.9	Unspecified open wound of eyeball
874.4	Penetrating wound of orbit with foreign body
918.1	Corneal laceration

CHEMICAL AND THERMAL INJURY

HISTORY

- Type of chemical (see Table 3-1), brand name, or product type of agent causing injury
- Time of injury and duration of exposure
- Prior attempts at irrigation
- Activity at time of injury
- Use of eye protection

FINDINGS ON EXAMINATION

- Facial skin and eyelid burns
- Conjunctival chemosis (Fig. 3-9)
- Conjunctival injection (conjunctiva may appear white and avascular if burn is severe)
- Corneal epithelial defects ranging from punctate staining to complete epithelial loss (Fig. 3-10)
- Loss of corneal clarity (localized corneal edema to complete corneal opacification)
- Aqueous cell and flare
- Increased or decreased intraocular pressure

EXAMINATION OUTLINE

- Examination should be deferred until adequate irrigation is complete and pH is neutral
- Check vision
- Slit lamp examination with instillation of fluorescein; evert upper eyelid and remove any debris or foreign material
- Check intraocular pressure

TABLE 3-1 **COMPONENTS OF COMMON SOURCES OF CHEMICAL INJURY**

Chemicals	Sources
Alkali	
Ammonia [NH_3]	Fertilizers, cleaning agents, refrigerants
Lye [$NaOH$]	Drain cleaners
Potassium hydroxide [KOH]	Caustic potash
Magnesium hydroxide [$MgOH$]	Sparklers, flares
Lime [$Ca(OH)_2$]	Plaster, mortar, cement, and whitewash (common in workplace, may leave particulate matter in conjunctival sac)
Acid	
Sulfuric acid [H_2SO_4]	Industrial cleaners, battery acid
Sulfurous acid [H_2SO_3]	Bleach, refrigerant
Hydrofluoric acid [HF]	Cleaning agent, etching of glass
Acetic acid [CH_3COOH]	Vinegar
Hydrochloric acid [HCl]	Cleaning agent
Organic	
Gasoline	
Acetone [C_3H_6O]	Fingernail polish, solvent
Benzene [C_6H_6]	Industrial solvent

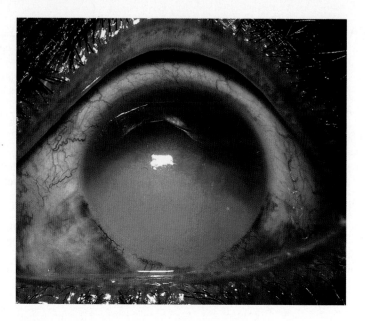

Figure 3-9 *Alkali injury to the eye causing an inferior epithelial defect (highlighted by the fluorescein dye), hemorrhage, and ischemia of the inferior conjunctiva.*

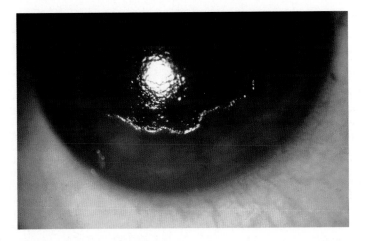

Figure 3-10 *Mild chemical injury. A central corneal abrasion from a splash of cleaning chemicals. The epithelial edge can be seen centrally. The epithelium on the inferior cornea is swollen and edematous. The conjunctiva is largely unaffected.*

TREATMENT

- Instill topical proparacaine or tetracaine to alleviate patient discomfort
- Immediate, copious irrigation with sterile saline or other isotonic solution for a minimum of 30 min
- Irrigation may be done as a drip, with plastic tubing, or with a squeeze bottle
- Consider use of an eyelid speculum or Morgan lens if the patient is unable to keep the eye open
- Check pH by touching litmus paper to conjunctival fornix; allow 5 to 10 min between irrigation and checking pH to allow for chemical equilibration; continue to lavage until pH is neutral
- Retained foreign bodies can cause persistently elevated pH; a cotton-tipped applicator moistened with topical anesthetic can be used to sweep particulate matter out of the conjunctival fornices; large particles can be removed with forceps

FOLLOW UP

- Severe chemical injury requires urgent ophthalmologic consultation
- Mild thermal injuries can be left unpatched with antibiotic ointment and seen in 1 to 2 days
- Prescribe a cycloplegic drop for ciliary body spasm and pain
- Oral analgesics as needed

PEARLS

- Normal pH of the conjunctival surface is between 6.8 and 7.4.
- All chemical injuries should be lavaged immediately. Defer further examination until pH has normalized.
- Extent of damage is dependent on concentration and pH of acid or base. (1) Alkali chemicals cause saponification of fat in cell membranes causing deep, rapid penetration of ocular tissues. (2) Acid burns coagulate and precipitate proteins, limiting the extent of ocular penetration. (3) Organic solvents primarily cause superficial epithelial damage and do not penetrate deeper ocular structures easily.
- Local poison control center may be helpful in determining specific properties of the materials involved.
- Thermal injury causes coagulation of epithelium, but usually does not injure deeper tissues.

ICD-9 CODES

940.0	Chemical burn of eyelids and periocular area
940.0	Other burns of cornea and conjunctival sac
940.1	Other burns of eyelids and periocular area
940.2	Alkaline burn of cornea and conjunctival sac
940.3	Acid chemical burn of cornea and conjunctival sac

HYPHEMA

HISTORY

- Type of trauma: blunt or sharp
- Sickle cell disease or trait
- Bleeding diathesis or liver disease
- Aspirin or anticoagulant use

FINDINGS ON EXAMINATION

SIGNS OF HYPHEMA

- Decreased vision
- Red blood cells layered in anterior chamber (Fig. 3-11)
- Free red blood cells in anterior chamber (called microhyphema when layered RBCs are absent)
- "Stunned" and poorly reactive pupil
- Increased or decreased intraocular pressure

CONCOMITANT SIGNS RELATED TO OCULAR TRAUMA

- Periorbital ecchymosis
- Lid lacerations
- Subconjunctival hemorrhage
- Corneal abrasion
- Iris sphincter tears
- Vossius' ring (pigment on anterior lens capsule) (Fig. 3-12)
- Iritis
- Lens subluxation or dislocation
- Ruptured globe
- Retinal detachment
- Vitreous hemorrhage

EXAMINATION OUTLINE

- Check visual acuity
- Check pupil reactivity
- Slit lamp examination with fluorescein dye
- Check intraocular pressure
- Dilated fundus examination
- Laboratory studies: Sickle prep and hemoglobin electrophoresis for all African American patients; PT/PTT and CBC if history suggests bleeding diathesis

TREATMENT

Treatment of hyphema is tailored to the cause and extent of the blood and any elevation of intraocular pressure (IOP). Patients usually require daily examinations, and patients are occasionally hospitalized to minimize activity.

- Atropine 1% BID—cycloplegic drugs help to minimize pain and discomfort
- Prednisolone acetate 1% QID
- Protective eye shield with holes
- Acetaminophen for pain
- Avoid aspirin and NSAIDs
- Bed rest with bathroom privileges
- Elevate head of bed

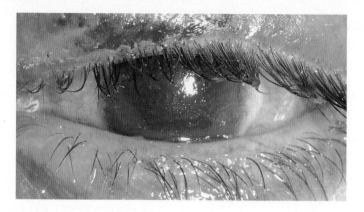

Figure 3-11 *Inferior hyphema in a car accident victim injured by airbag deployment. There is also periocular ecchymosis and irritation of the surface of the cornea.*

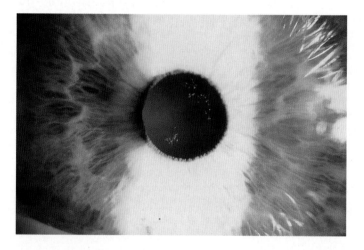

Figure 3-12 *Blunt trauma to the eye caused an imprint of iris pigment on the anterior lens capsule (Vossius' ring).*

- Aminocaproic acid, which may decrease the risk of rebleeding by inhibiting clot lysis and retraction, is recommended by some ophthalmologists; nausea, vomiting, and postural hypotension are common side effects of this medication, and patients must be hospitalized
- Treat increased intraocular pressure with aqueous suppressants, such as timolol and brimonidine (Alphagan); avoid latanaprost (Xalatan) or other prostaglandin analogues and pilocarpine, since these can exacerbate inflammation
- Anterior chamber washout—irrigation and removal of clotted blood from anterior chamber

FOLLOW UP

Patients with hyphema should be referred urgently for ophthalmologic evaluation.

ICD-9 CODE

364.41   Hyphema

CPT CODES

65815   Paracentesis of anterior chamber of eye with removal of blood, with or without irrigation and/or air injection

65930   Removal of blood clot, anterior segment eye

- An extensive hyphema can obscure other traumatic damage that becomes apparent as the blood clears.

- Rebleeding is a common complication of hyphema as the blood clot stabilizes and then retracts. Rebleeding usually occurs 2 to 5 days after the initial injury, and the hyphema after a rebleed is often more severe.

- Elevated intraocular pressure can occur in hyphema patients if red blood cells or breakdown products clog the trabecular meshwork and inhibit aqueous outflow. High IOP can lead to optic nerve damage, ischemic vascular events in the retina, and corneal blood staining. Surgical evacuation of the blood may be needed.

- Sickle cell patients, particularly with HbAS and HbSC subtypes, are at special risk for IOP elevation as sickled blood cells are more likely than normal RBCs to obstruct the trabecular meshwork. Avoid oral and topical carbonic anhydrase inhibitors (acetazolamide [Diamox], methazolamide [Neptazane], brinzolamide [Azopt] and dorzolmide [Trusopt]) because these can cause a metabolic acidosis and worsen sickling.

LENS SUBLUXATION OR DISLOCATION

HISTORY

- Symptoms of decreased visual acuity, occasionally monocular diplopia
- Blunt or penetrating trauma
- In absence of trauma, inquire about history of Marfan's syndrome, homocystinuria, Weill–Marchesani syndrome, or family history thereof

FINDINGS ON EXAMINATION

- Iris sphincter tears
- Vossius' ring—round imprint of iris pigment on anterior lens capsule (Fig. 3-12)
- Cataract—specifically stellate opacity resulting secondary to trauma
- Iridodonesis—quivering of the iris occurring with eye movement
- Phacodonesis—quivering of the lens occurring with head or eye movement or blinking
- Edge of lens visible through dilated pupil (subluxation) (Fig. 3-13)
- Lens not visible through pupillary aperture (total dislocation) (Fig. 3-14)
- Prolapse of vitreous into anterior chamber

EXAMINATION OUTLINE

- Check visual acuity
- Check pupils and reactivity
- Slit lamp examination—look particularly at edge of pupil and lens
- Dilated fundus examination for retinal detachments or lens dislocation into vitreous

TREATMENT

In the setting of trauma, lens dislocation warrants urgent ophthalmologic consultation as other ocular structures are frequently injured

FOLLOW UP

As determined by ophthalmologist.

ICD-9 CODE

379.32   Subluxation of lens

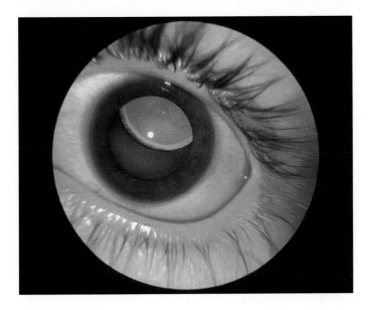

Figure 3-13 *Superotemporal subluxation of the lens in the left eye of a patient with Marfan's syndrome.*

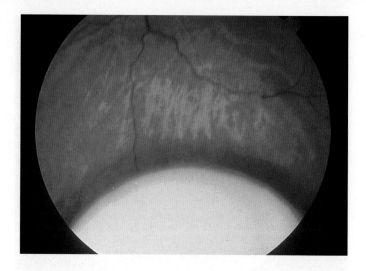

Figure 3-14 *White, cataractous lens dislocated into the vitreous cavity.*

INTRAOCULAR FOREIGN BODY (IOFB)

HISTORY

- Activity at time of injury: hammering, grinding, use of power tools, gunplay
- Material composition of presumed foreign body (e.g., iron, wood, glass)
- Tetanus immunization history

FINDINGS ON EXAMINATION

- Lid lacerations
- Conjunctival laceration
- Subconjunctival hemorrhage may be present 360° around corneal limbus
- Corneal laceration with or without extrusion of ocular contents
- Corneal edema
- Round or irregular pupil
- Deep or shallow anterior chamber
- Foreign body in anterior chamber or retina (Fig. 3-15)
- Decreased intraocular pressure
- Hyphema
- Restriction of ocular motility
- Lens dislocation (edge of lens visible through pupil)
- Cataract
- Vitreous hemorrhage
- Commotio retinae
- Retinal detachment

EXAMINATION OUTLINE

- Check visual acuity
- Check pupils for afferent pupillary defect
- Test ocular motility
- Slit lamp examination using fluorescein dye
- Avoid maneuvers that could apply pressure on the globe and cause further extrusion of intraocular contents
- Seidel test for leakage of intraocular fluid
- Dilated fundus examination
- CT scan of head and orbits is essential in the evaluation of presumed IOFB; axial and coronal images with thin (2 to 3 mm) slices are preferable
- MRI is contraindicated when metal foreign bodies are suspected
- B-scan ultrasonography may help identify glass or metallic foreign bodies

TREATMENT

- Many cases of penetrating ocular injury will require operative exploration and repair
- Proper assessment and management in the emergency department can assure proper preoperative preparation and prevent further damage to the eye
- Protect eye with metal shield, avoid placing pressure on the globe by affixing tape to the cheek and forehead
- Broad spectrum antibiotics:
    - vancomycin, 1 g IV every 12 h
    - ceftazidime, 1 g IV every 8 h
- Antiemetics to prevent increase in intraocular pressure caused by Valsalva maneuver
- Transport patient with head of bed elevated
- Patients with presumed or apparent penetrating ocular injuries should be evaluated by an ophthalmologist on an emergent basis

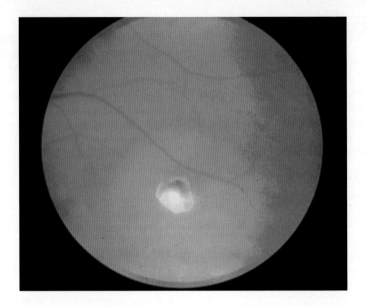

Figure 3-15 *Steel foreign body embedded in retina with surrounding localized retinal detachment (whitish circular area around foreign body).*

- Extensive bullous subconjunctival hemorrhage or very low intraocular pressure is suggestive of scleral rupture.

- It is possible to have a penetrating ocular injury with no apparent damage to the cornea or conjunctiva. A foreign body may pass through the lids and sclera without interrupting the conjunctiva.

- Copper, iron, and steel typically cause severe inflammatory reactions in the eye. Vegetable matter can elicit severe inflammation and harbor virulent bacteria.

ICD-9 CODES

360.50 Foreign body, magnetic, intraocular, unspecified
360.60 Foreign body, intraocular, unspecified

871.5 Penetration of eyeball with magnetic foreign body
871.6 Penetration of eyeball with (nonmagnetic) foreign body

CPT CODES

65205 Removal of foreign body, external eye, conjunctival superficial
65210 Removal of foreign body, external eye, conjunctival embedded
65220 Removal of foreign body, corneal, without slit lamp
65222 Removal of foreign body, corneal, with slit lamp
65235 Removal of foreign body, intraocular, from anterior chamber or lens
65260 Removal of foreign body, from posterior segment, magnetic extraction, anterior or posterior route
65265 Removal of foreign body, from posterior segment, nonmagnetic extraction, anterior or posterior route

TRAUMATIC RETINAL DAMAGE

Includes the following entities:

- Commotio retinae
- Retinal detachment
- Giant retinal tear
- Traumatic macular hole
- Preretinal hemorrhage

HISTORY

- Blunt ocular trauma
- Decrease in visual acuity
- Flashing lights
- New onset of floaters

FINDINGS ON EXAMINATION

Decreased visual acuity if macula is involved with any of the conditions.

COMMOTIO RETINAE

- Localized or widespread areas of confluent retinal whitening, usually located peripherally
- Partial or absolute scotomas on visual fields corresponding to affected area

RETINAL DETACHMENT AND GIANT RETINAL TEAR (FIG. 3-16)

- Whitish wrinkled retina thrown into folds
- Pigment or red blood cells in vitreous
- Retinal tear may be found adjacent to a chorioretinal scar
- Peripheral shadow or dark curtain over vision

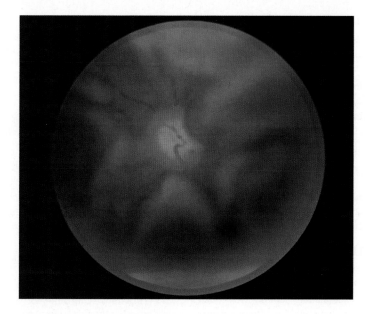

Figure 3-16 *Total retinal detachment with the retina thrown into gentle folds around the optic nerve.*

TRAUMATIC MACULAR HOLE (FIG. 3-17)

- Decrease in vision often worse than 20/200
- Partial or full thickness retinal defect in macula with the underlying choroid visible
- Cuff of subretinal fluid surrounding the hole
- Central scotoma, interferes with reading
- Discrete yellowish deposits (drusen) in center of macular hole

PRERETINAL HEMORRHAGE (FIG. 3-18)

- Decreased vision, especially if blood overlies macula
- Boat-shaped hemorrhage
- Red blood cells scattered in vitreous
- Scotomas correspond to location of blood

EXAMINATION OUTLINE

- Check vision
- Check pupils
- Slit lamp examination looking for other signs ocular trauma and for vitreous debris
- Check IOP (can be decreased in retinal detachments)
- Dilated fundus examination

TREATMENT

- Commotio retinae: refer to retinal specialist within a week or two; often resolves spontaneously, may have residual visual field loss
- Retinal tear/detachment, giant retinal tear; and preretinal hemorrhage: refer urgently to ophthalmologist for evaluation and management
- Traumatic macular hole: Refer to ophthalmologist in a timely manner

PEARLS

- Patients with pigment or red blood cells in the vitreous are significantly more likely to have a retinal tear or detachment.

- Traumatic macular holes have been known to close spontaneously with restoration of good vision.

- Other causes of preretinal hemorrhages include following a Valsalva maneuver, severe chest trauma (Purtcher's syndrome), or a subarachnoid hemorrhage (Terson's syndrome).

ICD-9 CODES

361.0	Retinal detachment with retinal defect
362.54	Macular cyst, hole, or pseudohole
362.81	Retinal hemorrhage
362.82	Retinal edema
921.3	Commotio retinae
921.3	Contusion of eyeball

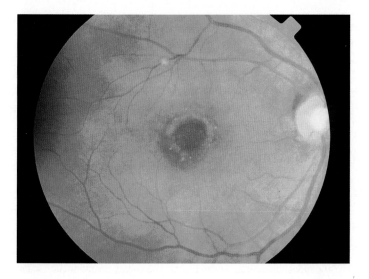

Figure 3-17 *Full thickness macular hole. Note the circular cuff of retinal elevation and the central hole. Vision in this case is 20/400.*

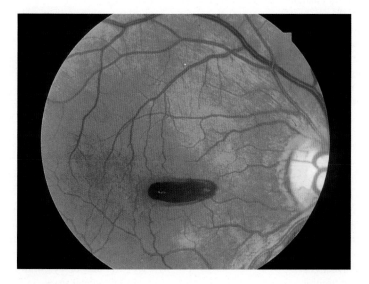

Figure 3-18 *Oval preretinal hemorrhage. The blood is trapped between the vitreous and the retinal surface.*

RUPTURED GLOBE AND SCLERAL RUPTURE

HISTORY

- Mechanism of trauma—sharp or blunt injury
- Prior ocular surgery
- Prior ocular injury
- Prior tetanus immunization

FINDINGS ON EXAMINATION

- Decreased vision
- Extensive subconjunctival hemorrhage
- Limitation of ocular motility
- Afferent pupillary defect
- Extrusion of intraocular contents (Fig. 3-19)
- Periorbital ecchymosis
- Maxillofacial fractures including orbital blowout fractures
- Corneal abrasion
- Hyphema
- Decreased intraocular pressure
- Shallow anterior chamber when compared to fellow eye
- Irregular pupil
- Iris sphincter tears
- Lens dislocation
- Vitreous hemorrhage
- Commotio retinae (areas of retinal whitening); see also section "Traumatic Retinal Damage"
- Retinal breaks, tears, or detachment
- Choroidal rupture (Fig. 3-20)
- Traumatic optic neuropathy

EXAMINATION OUTLINE

- If rupture is suspected, it is appropriate to defer further examination until an ophthalmologist is available; cover eye with a metal or plastic shield to keep pressure off the globe
- Check visual acuity
- Check pupil reactivity
- Check ocular motility
- Slit lamp examination
- Seidel test
- Check intraocular pressure; defer if rupture is suspected
- Dilated fundus examination
- CT scan of head and orbits; axial and coronal images with thin (2 to 3 mm) slices are preferable; MRI is contraindicated when metal intraocular foreign bodies are suspected

TREATMENT

- Surgical exploration and repair is usually indicated for patients suspected of having a ruptured globe.
- If open globe injury is suspected, cover the eye with a shield. Avoid placing pressure on the eye.
- While awaiting ophthalmologic assessment patients should be NPO in case surgery is necessary. Antiemetic agents, to prevent increases in intraocular pressure from a Valsalva maneuver, should be considered. Elevate head of bed, shield globe.

FOLLOW UP

Open globe injuries require immediate ophthalmic attention.

PEARLS

- Extensive bullous subconjunctival hemorrhage is highly suggestive of ruptured globe.

- If ruptured globe is suspected, further examination should be deferred until the patient can be examined in an operating room.

ICD-9 CODES

871.1   Ocular laceration with prolapse of intraocular tissue
871.2   Rupture of eye with partial loss of intraocular tissue
871.9   Unspecified open wound of eyeball
921.3   Contusion of eyeball

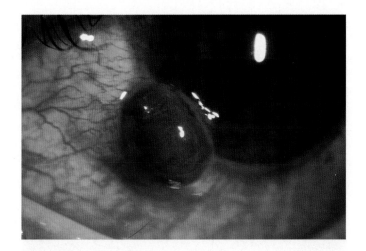

Figure 3-19 *Ruptured globe with prolapse of iris through the wound and an irregularly shaped pupil.*

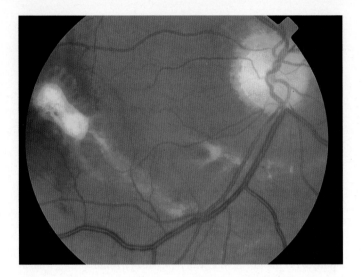

Figure 3-20 *Healed choroidal rupture appearing as an arc-shaped break in the choroid allowing the underlying yellow-white sclera to be visible. Fibrosis and scarring also occur at these sites. The rupture through the macula often results in poor central visual acuity.*

TRAUMATIC OPTIC NEUROPATHY (TON)

HISTORY

- Direct severe trauma to head, eye, or periocular region
- Alteration of consciousness

FINDINGS ON EXAMINATION

- Dramatically decreased vision
- Afferent pupillary defect
- Normal appearing optic nerve in the acute phase
- Optic nerve head pallor and atrophy in chronic phase

LESS COMMON SIGNS

- Optic nerve head swelling
- Optic nerve and retinal hemorrhages
- Central retinal artery occlusion
- Central retinal vein occlusion
- Constriction of visual field

EXAMINATION OUTLINE

- Check vision
- Check pupils for afferent pupillary defect
- Assess visual fields by confrontation
- Check color vision
- Dilated fundus examination to rule out other retinal pathology
- Computed tomography of head and orbits with concentration on bony optic canal

TREATMENT

- Treatment of TON is controversial
- High-dose IV steroids and optic canal decompression surgery are the mainstays of treatment

FOLLOW UP

- Prognosis for recovery of vision is guarded
- Patients suspected of having TON should be referred urgently for ophthalmologic and/or neurosurgical evaluation

PEARLS

- In the absence of severe retinal pathology, an afferent papillary defect is highly suggestive of optic nerve pathology.

- With head trauma, concussive forces can be directed to the optic canal. The optic nerve can be damaged secondary to compression from hemorrhage or edema or lacerated by fractured bone.

- Patients with traumatic optic neuropathy often have other head and neck injuries. Neurosurgical and head and neck specialists should be alerted.

ICD-9 CODES

377.49   Compression of optic nerve
377.42   Hemorrhage in optic nerve sheath
950.0   Optic nerve injury

LID LACERATION

HISTORY

- Time course—how long ago did the injury happen?
- Method of injury? Activity at time of injury?
- Laceration caused by what object? (metal, glass, wood, dog bite)
- Possibility of foreign body in wound or within the eye? (if the object was a sharp projectile or could fragment easily)
- Most recent tetanus vaccination?
- Was the injury caused by an animal or human bite? Does the patient know the owner of the animal? Any abnormal animal behavior? Contact the local animal care department

FINDINGS ON EXAMINATION

COMMON FINDINGS (FIGS. 3-21 AND 3-22)

- Laceration involving the superficial lid, lid margin, or deeper lid exposing septal fat
- Periorbital/lid edema
- Periorbital/lid ecchymosis
- Subconjunctival hemorrhage/injection
- Conjunctival laceration
- Corneal abrasion/laceration

LESS COMMON FINDINGS

- Ruptured globe—shallow anterior chamber, protrusion of intraocular material
- Blood in anterior chamber (hyphema)

EXAMINATION OUTLINE

- Does the wound involve the lid margin?
- Does the wound involve the lacrimal drainage system?
- Is there septal fat protruding?
- Check extent of wound—look for any missing tissue
- Rough check of visual acuity
- Check reactivity of pupil with penlight

- Check for a ruptured globe—shallow anterior chamber, 360° subconjunctival hemorrhage, deep corneal foreign body, soft globe
- Check extraocular motility (decreased upgaze may signal involvement of superior rectus)
- Diplopia in any of the fields of gaze? (also may indicate involvement of ocular muscles)
- Check orbicularis function by having patient close the eyes tightly
- Look for ptosis (droopy eyelid), which may signal involvement of levator aponeurosis of upper eyelid
- Check the wound for a foreign body (this can be done after local anesthesia is administered)
- CT (axial/coronal) of orbit and brain in cases of significant orbital trauma or when a retained foreign body or ruptured globe are suspected

TREATMENT

- Tetanus prophylaxis if needed
- For minor lacerations, surgical repair
- Refer to ophthalmologist for repair in operating room
  - if associated with ruptured globe; involves lacrimal drainage system or levator aponeurosis of upper eyelid (ptosis present) or superior rectus muscle (decreased supraduction and orbital fat exposed)
  - if avulsed medial canthal tendon present (abnormal amount of laxity over medial canthus), and extensive tissue loss (more than two thirds of eyelid)
- For wounds that need to be repaired in the operating room, keep the wound moist with gauze soaked in sterile saline until the repair (which should be done within 48 h)
- If the laceration involves the eyelid margin, call an ophthalmologist
- Delay repair for heavily contaminated wounds and animal/human bites

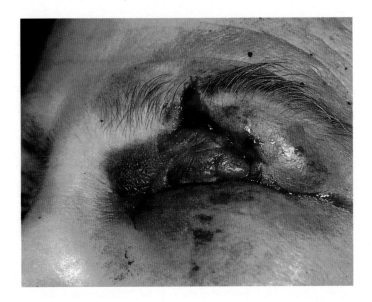

Figure 3-21 *Deep brow laceration to the left upper lid not involving the lid margin. Repaired with deep Vicryl sutures and nylon sutures for skin closure (Table 3-2).*

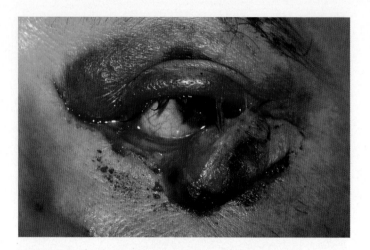

Figure 3-22 *Lid laceration of the right eye involving the inferior canalicular system. Reconstructed by ophthalmologist in operating room with silicone intubation of the lacrimal drainage system and reattachment of the lid to the medial canthus.*

TABLE 3-2   TECHNIQUE FOR REPAIR OF MINOR LACERATIONS

- Instill topical proparacaine drops
- Clean periocular area with povidone iodine solution (Betadine); *do not use iodine scrub solution around the eye*
- Local subcutaneous anesthesia (2% lidocaine with epinephrine)
- Copiously irrigate wound with saline in a syringe
- Explore wound for foreign bodies and remove them
- Debridement of infected or necrotic tissue (remove as little as possible)
- Protective eye shell over the cornea
- For superficial cuts parallel to the skin creases, steri-strips can be used to reapproximate skin edges
- Vicryl 6-0 for deep sutures but do not pass through the posterior part of the eyelid
- Nylon 6-0 or 7-0 or Vicryl 6-0 or 7-0 suture for skin and orbicularis in an interrupted fashion (make sure to evert the skin edges)
- Ice compresses TID
- Keep the head of the bed elevated 30° for 48 h
- Antibiotic ointment BID
- Systemic antibiotics (dicloxacillin or cephalexin) if contamination suspected (consider penicillin V for animal/human bites)
- Massage the wound at 3 to 4 weeks post-repair to prevent contracture

FOLLOW UP

- Refer urgently for ruptured globe, laceration needing repair in the OR, or lacerations involving the lid margin
- Eyelid sutures need to be removed in 4 to 6 days if not absorbable
- Eyelid margin sutures need to be left in place for 10 to 14 days

PEARLS

- Do not shave the eyebrows for brow lacerations as they may not grow back.

- Vicryl (or other absorbable suture) can be used to close the skin if compliance is an issue, but results in more scarring

- If the laceration involves the lid margin, call an ophthalmologist. If none is available, pass 6-0 silk through the gray line of the eyelid margin to approximate the edges, and then pass another either anterior or posterior to the gray line. Leave the ends of the suture long and secure to the eyelid skin so they do not irritate the cornea.

ICD-9 CODES

870.0   Lid laceration involving skin and periocular area
870.1   Full thickness lid laceration
870.2   Lid laceration involving the lacrimal system

CPT CODES

67930   Partial thickness eyelid wound repair
67935   Full thickness eyelid wound repair
67938   Removal of embedded eyelid foreign body
12001–12007 Simple repair of superficial wounds
12051–12057 Layered closure of facial wounds

BLOW-OUT FRACTURES

HISTORY

DEFINITION Fracture involving the orbital floor (maxillary bone) but sparing the orbital rim; also usually involving the posterior medial floor (weakest point).

- History of recent trauma? By what?
- Time course—when did the trauma happen?
- Is the swelling worse after nose blowing?

FINDINGS ON EXAMINATION

- Enophthalmos or exophthalmos (eye sunken in or protruding out)
- Limited eye motility (especially with vertical movement) secondary to entrapment of ocular muscles, muscle contusion, or nerve damage (Fig. 3-23)
- Binocular double vision (especially in upgaze or downgaze)
- Pain (especially with vertical ocular movements)
- Eyelid swelling (worse after nose blowing) with subcutaneous emphysema
- Infraorbital paresthesias, hypesthesia of the gums and upper lip
- Palpable step-off of bony orbital rim

- Point tenderness
- Ptosis (droopy eyelid)
- Nosebleed

EXAMINATION OUTLINE

- Visual acuity
- Check reactivity of pupils
- Palpate for step-off, point tenderness, subcutaneous crepitus
- Open lids and check for ruptured globe (shallow anterior chamber, 360° subconjunctival hemorrhage)
- Check globe with slit lamp for hyphema, traumatic mydriasis, traumatic iritis, lens subluxation
- Check ocular motility and look closely for any restriction (may be secondary to entrapment or edema)
- Double vision in any of the fields of gaze? (also may be a sign of entrapment)
- Check infraorbital sensation and compare with other side
- Check for proptosis (protruding eye)
- CT of the orbits and brain (axial and coronal sections) to rule out muscle entrapment, check size of fracture, visualize air trapped in the tissues, and identify nasal wall or orbital roof fracture (Figs. 3-23 and 3-24)

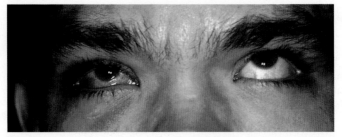

A

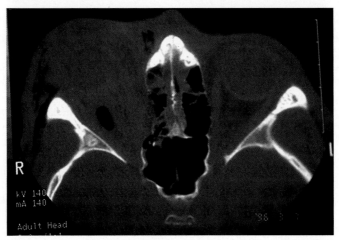

B

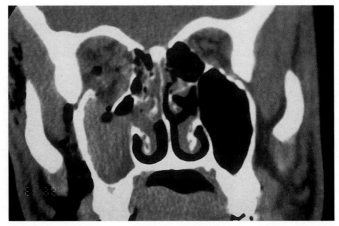

C

Figure 3-23 *A. Right inferior and medial floor fracture with marked restriction in upgaze. B. Axial CT sections showing the right medial wall fracture with air in the orbit. C. Coronal CT sections showing the right medial wall fracture and the largely displaced floor fracture. Note the loss of ethmoid space, opacified maxillary sinus, and air in the orbit.*

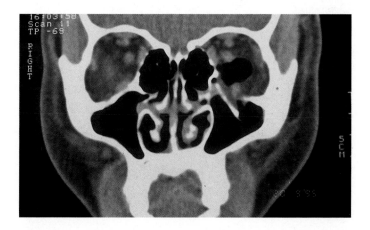

Figure 3-24 *Left inferior rectus entrapment secondary to the left inferior floor fracture. Air can also be seen in the center of the orbit inferior to the optic nerve.*

TREATMENT

- Nasal decongestants for 2 weeks
- Oral cephalexin (Keflex) or erythromycin for 10 to 14 d
- No nose blowing
- Ice to area the first 24 to 48 h to reduce swelling
- Elevation of head of bed
- Pain management
- Avoid anticoagulants and aspirin for 14 d
- Surgical repair immediately for muscle entrapment seen on CT
- Surgical repair at 7 to 14 d if persistent double vision in primary position or when reading, enophthalmos, or large fracture (involving more than two thirds of floor)
- Neurosurgical consult for roof fractures

FOLLOW UP

- Consult Neurosurgery urgently if a roof fracture is present or if the fracture extends to the optic canal
- Refer urgently if muscle entrapment is seen on CT
- 1 to 2 weeks with ophthalmologist to look for persistent double vision or enophthalmos after edema has subsided
- 1 to 2 weeks with ophthalmologist to check for accessory damage from blunt trauma such as angle recession and retinal detachment
- Warn patient of signs of retinal detachment (flashes, many floaters, curtain coming over the vision) and orbital cellulitis (pain with eye movement, fever, increasing erythema, and edema)

PEARLS

- The initial restriction in ocular motility is often secondary to orbital edema. If no entrapment is seen on CT, re-evaluate in 1 week after much of the edema has subsided.

- If a child, consider child abuse.

ICD-9 CODES

802.6	Closed blow-out fracture
802.7	Open blow-out fracture
802.8	Fracture involving other facial bones

Chapter 4

CONJUNCTIVA

KAMBIZ NEGAHBAN

BACTERIAL CONJUNCTIVITIS

HISTORY

DURATION   (1) Hyperacute (within 12 to 24 h), (2) acute (less than 4 weeks), (3) chronic (greater than 4 weeks).

BILATERALITY   Acute and chronic bacterial conjunctivitis are usually unilateral

TYPE OF DISCHARGE   Usually presents as mild to moderate mucoid or mucopurulent discharge.

FOREIGN BODY SENSATION   Mild scratchiness and irritation is typical. If itching component is prominent, suspect allergic causes.

PHOTOPHOBIA   Mild degree is typical. Suspect a uveitic component if photophobia is out of proportion to findings.

FLASHES AND FLOATERS   Consider retinal pathology (e.g., retinal detachment, posterior vitreous detachment, retinal breaks) if history consists of acute flashes or floaters (see Chapter 9).

SEXUAL HISTORY   A history of vaginitis, cervicitis, or urethritis may be present in chronic cases.

FINDINGS ON EXAMINATION (SEE FIG. 4-1)

- Red injected eye: conjunctivitis involves conjunctival and episcleral vessels; sclera is not involved (Table 4-1)
- Purulent and mucopurulent discharge
- Eyelid swelling
- Chemosis: edema of the conjunctiva
- Preauricular lymphadenopathy: more common with viral causes

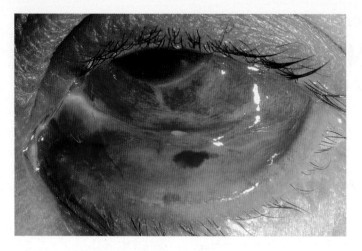

Figure 4-1 *Hyperacute conjunctivitis as evident by copious mucopurulent discharge, conjunctival edema, and hemorrhage. Organisms such as* Neisseria *should always be considered.*

TABLE 4-1   DIFFERENTIAL DIAGNOSES OF RED EYE

- Conjunctivitis
- Dry eyes and keratoconjunctivitis sicca
- Iritis and uveitis
- Blepharitis
- Injected pterygium and pingueculum
- Subconjunctival hemorrhage
- Dacryocystitis and canaliculitis
- Acute angle closure glaucoma
- Episcleritis
- Scleritis

EXAMINATION OUTLINE

- Instill a drop of proparacaine (topical anesthetic) if patient is unable to open eye to cooperate secondary to pain; check corneal sensation before if viral causes (e.g. herpes) suspected
- Check visual acuity; a near visual acuity card is useful if patient is bedridden
- Check reactivity of pupils; during this part of the examination, observe patient's subjective photophobia to your light source
- Slit lamp examination; look for papillae (dilated, telangiectatic conjunctival blood vessels appearing as dots) or follicles (raised focal lymphoid nodules) on the inferior palpebral conjunctiva; follicles indicate chronic inclusion conjunctivitis or viral causes
- Check for cells and flare in the anterior chamber with a small, narrow slit beam
- Instill a drop of fluorescein dye or touch conjunctival surface with a moistened fluorescein strip and examine with cobalt blue light
- If severe, consider conjunctival swabbing for bacterial cultures (blood and chocolate agars) and Gram's and Giemsa stain; for a follicular conjunctivitis, consider conjunctival swabs for viral or chlamydial cultures
- Check for preauricular lymphadenopathy

TREATMENT

HYPERACUTE CONJUNCTIVITIS AND GONOCOCCAL CONJUNCTIVITIS If gram-negative intracellular diplococci seen on Gram's stain, administer ceftriaxone 1 g IM as single dose, and refer to an ophthalmologist on an emergency basis.

ACUTE CONJUNCTIVITIS If no contraindications present, start with topical broad-spectrum antibiotic therapy for 5 to 7 days; examples are:

- Trimethoprim–polymixin QID
- Ofloxacin QID
- Ciprofloxacin QID
- Bacitracin–erythromycin ointment TID

CHRONIC CONJUNCTIVITIS Chlamydial inclusion conjunctivitis (Giemsa stain showing basophilic intracytoplasmic inclusion bodies); treat with:

- Oral antibiotics: doxycycline 100 mg po BID; tetracycline 250 to 500 mg po QID; erythromycin 250 to 500 mg po BID *or* clarithromycin 250 to 500 mg po BID
- Topical ointments: erythromycin, tetracycline, or sulfacetamide 2 to 3 times per day for 2 to 3 weeks

FOLLOW UP

HYPERACUTE CONJUNCTIVITIS Urgently with ophthalmologist.

ACUTE OR CHRONIC CONJUNCTIVITIS In 2 days, and then 5 to 7 days until conjunctivitis resolves. If no resolution is seen, refer to an ophthalmologist for evaluation on an urgent basis. Refer immediately for hyperpurulent conjunctivitis.

ICD-9 CODES

077.0	Adult inclusion conjunctivitis
372.0	Acute conjunctivitis
372.04	Mucopurulent conjunctivitis
372.12	Chronic follicular conjunctivitis
372.20	Blepharoconjunctivitis, unspecified

VIRAL CONJUNCTIVITIS

HISTORY

DURATION AND LATERALITY Usually acute (less than 4 weeks), and bilateral (generally starts in one eye, and the fellow eye is affected several days later).

TYPE OF DISCHARGE Watery discharge with scant whitish mucus.

SYMPTOMS

- History of a recent upper respiratory tract infection *OR* contact with someone who is suffering from a red eye
- Itching, burning and foreign body sensation; can have mild photophobia
- Febrile if associated with pharyngoconjunctival fever

FINDINGS ON EXAMINATION

COMMON

- Red and swollen eyelids (Fig. 4-2)
- Palpable preauricular lymph node

- Inferior palpebral conjunctival follicles (focal lymphoid nodules with accessory vascularization)
- Watery mucous discharge

LESS COMMON

- Pinpoint subconjunctival petechial hemorrhages (Fig. 4-3)
- Membrane or pseudomembrane formation (inflammatory coagulum on the conjunctival surface)
- Subepithelial corneal infiltrates (Fig. 4-4) usually occur about 1 to 2 weeks after the onset of conjunctivitis and appear as white fluffy opacities in the subepithelial layer of the cornea

UNCOMMON

Should prompt further investigation for other causes

- Corneal ulcer (see Chapter 5)
- Anterior chamber cells
- Hypopyon: layering of white blood cells in the anterior chamber

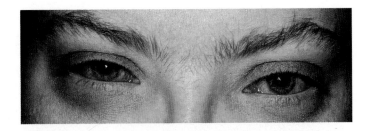

Figure 4-2 *A 25-year old patient with bilateral redness, eyelid swelling, foreign body sensation, and watery discharge caused by adenovirus (epidemic keratoconjunctivitis, EKC).*

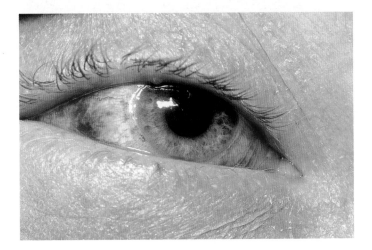

Figure 4-3 *Conjunctival injection and subconjunctival petechial hemorrhages are more commonly seen with EKC than with other viral infections.*

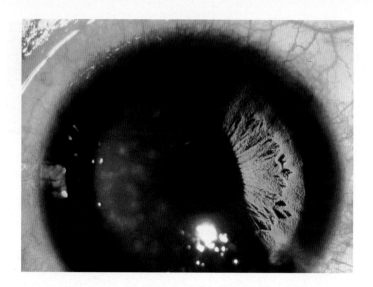

Figure 4-4 *Diffusely scattered subepithelial infiltrates appear as the viral infection is resolving and represent an inflammatory reaction to viral antigens in the corneal stroma.*

EXAMINATION OUTLINE

- Rough check of visual acuity
- Instill a drop of proparacaine (topical anesthetic) if patient is unable to open eye to cooperate because of pain
- Check for pre-auricular lymphadenopathy
- Slit lamp examination
- Examine the inferior palpebral conjunctiva carefully for follicles (a common sign for viral conjunctivitis)
- Instill a drop of fluorescein dye or touch conjunctival surface with moistened fluorescein strip and examine with cobalt blue light
- Diffuse pattern of coarse punctate staining is consistent with a viral etiology
- Send viral cultures or adenovirus DFA if the etiology is still unclear

TREATMENT

- Treatment is usually supportive since viral conjunctivitis is usually self-limited
- Preservative-free artificial tears 4 to 6 times per day for lubrication of the ocular surface
- If itching is a severe component, consider using naphazoline/pheniramine drops QID
- Cool compresses several times per day for 1 to 3 weeks as needed for comfort
- Advise patient that this condition is very contagious and he or she should avoid touching the eyes, use disposable tissues, and limit contact with other people for 10 to 12 days from the day of onset; frequent handwashing decreases the rate of infection

FOLLOW UP

- Refer to an ophthalmologist if a membrane or a pseudomembrane is seen
- Patient may be safely followed up in 1 to 2 weeks, or sooner if the condition worsens
- Refer to an ophthalmologist if the condition does not resolve after 3 weeks or patient has atypical symptoms

PEARLS

- Viral conjunctivitis can worsen initially in the first 4 to 7 days.

- Etiology is usually adenovirus (subtypes 8, 11, 19). If the patient is from tropical regions of the world, acute hemorrhagic conjunctivitis caused by enterovirus or coxsackievirus is possible.

ICD-9 CODES

077.0	Viral keratoconjunctivitis NOS
077.1	Epidemic keratoconjunctivitis
372.02	Acute follicular conjunctivitis
372.12	Chronic follicular conjunctivitis

ALLERGIC CONJUNCTIVITIS

HISTORY

DURATION AND LATERALITY Usually short-lived (rapid development after exposure) and bilateral.

MEDICAL HISTORY Frequent in patients with history of atopy, allergic rhinitis, or asthma.

ALLERGY HISTORY Pollen, dust mites, animal dander, etc.

SYMPTOMS

- Itching: hallmark symptom
- Watery discharge
- Red eye

FINDINGS ON EXAMINATION

COMMON

- Red eye
- Stringy, white discharge
- Eyelid swelling
- Chemosis: edema of the conjunctiva (Fig. 4-5)
- No preauricular lymphadenopathy
- Conjunctival papillae (dilated telangiectatic conjunctival blood vessels, varying from dotlike changes to enlarged tufts) (see Fig. 4-6)

LESS COMMON

- Punctate epithelial keratopathy
- Photophobia

UNCOMMON
Should prompt further investigation for other causes.

- Anterior chamber cells
- Corneal ulcer and infiltrate
- Mucopurulent and purulent discharge

EXAMINATION OUTLINE

- Rough check of visual acuity
- Instill a drop of proparacaine (topical anesthetic) if patient is unable to open eye to cooperate because of pain
- Slit lamp examination: examine the inferior palpebral conjunctiva carefully to detect papillae (see above); evert the upper lid to detect any papillary changes
- Instill a drop of fluorescein eye or touch conjunctival surface with moistened fluorescein strip and examine with cobalt blue light; alternatively, the cobalt blue feature of a direct ophthalmoscope may be used if a slit lamp is not available
- Examine the corneal surface for any uptake or staining with fluorescein; typically, there is no staining.

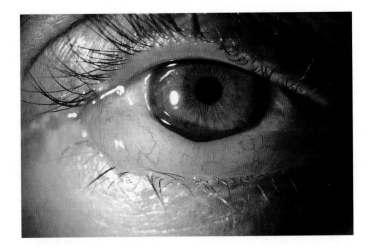

Figure 4-5 *Classic chemosis—after exposure to an allergan (e.g., cat dander), the eyes get extremely itchy and the conjunctiva swells with a clear, serous transudate.*

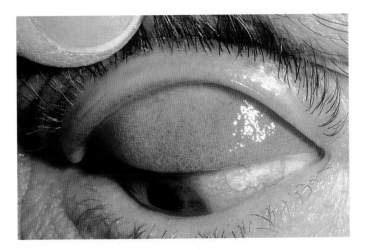

Figure 4-6 *Conjunctival papillae under the upper eyelid are a non-specific response to irritation causing dilation of the fine pinpoint tarsal blood vessels.*

TREATMENT

- Encourage the patient to eliminate the offending agent; thorough cleaning of carpets, linen, and bedding can be helpful for removing accumulated allergens
- Treatment is based on the severity of patient's symptoms
- Cool compresses several times per day
- Consider following topical treatment depending on severity: preservative-free artificial tears 4 to 6 times per day; chilling tears will provide additional relief when instilled; artificial tears can be combined with a combined vasoconstrictor/antihistamine (e.g., naphazoline/pheniramine) agent QID
- Consider oral or topical antihistamines in moderate to severe cases

FOLLOW UP

- Patients are instructed to return in 2 weeks for follow up
- Refer to an ophthalmologist
  - if severe allergic conjunctivitis requires using topical steroids
  - if there is significant visual loss or atypical symptoms

PEARLS

- Itching is a hallmark sign of allergic conjunctivitis. Rubbing of the eyelids causes degranulation of the mast cells and eosinophils, exacerbating the itching and irritation.

- Many patients may be self-medicating before they see their physician. Using topical vasoconstrictors, alone or in combination with antihistamines, may provide acute symptomatic relief. However, their use for more than 5 to 7 consecutive days may predispose to rebound phenomenon characterized by tachyphylaxis (decreased effectiveness of medication with increased use) and rebound injection.

ICD-9 CODES

372.05   Acute atopic conjunctivitis
372.13   Vernal conjunctivitis
372.14   Chronic allergic conjunctivitis

SUBCONJUNCTIVAL HEMORRHAGE

HISTORY

- Activity: history of Valsalva, heavy lifting, coughing, or straining secondary to constipation
- Trauma history or eye rubbing
- Hypertension
- Bleeding diathesis and disorder or anticoagulation
- Medications: elicit any history of aspirin or coumadin use
- Idiopathic

FINDINGS ON EXAMINATION

- Usually asymptomatic
- Red eye with occasional foreign body sensation
- Bright red or dark maroon blood underneath the conjunctiva, often sectoral (Fig. 4-7)
- Brightness of red blood appears much worse than the actual condition
- If there is 360° of subconjunctival hemorrhage or history of trauma, *must rule out ruptured globe*

EXAMINATION OUTLINE

- Instill a drop of proparacaine (topical anesthetic) if patient is unable to open eye to cooperate because of pain; suspect other coexisting etiologies if severe pain or photophobia
- Rough check of visual acuity
- Check reactivity of the pupils and rule out an afferent pupillary defect
- Slit lamp examination
- Suspect a ruptured globe if subconjunctival hemorrhage involves 360°
- If the patient has a history of recurrent subconjunctival hemorrhage of bleeding diathesis, consider ordering a bleeding time, prothrombin time, partial thromboplastin, and complete blood count with platelets and protein C and S

TREATMENT

- No treatment is required
- Artificial tear drops QID prn if the patient is symptomatic
- Consider stopping anticoagulants if there are no contraindications

FOLLOW UP

- Gradual clearing in 1 to 2 weeks
- Referral to patient's primary care doctor if there is poorly controlled hypertension or to rule out a bleeding diathesis

ICD-9 CODES

372.72   Conjunctival (subconjunctival) hemorrhage

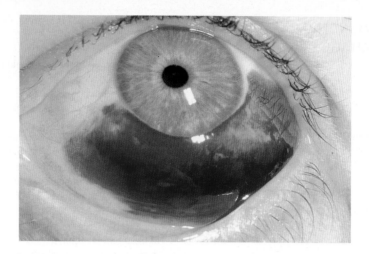

Figure 4-7   *Inferior subconjunctiival hemorrhage. Note that the remainder of the conjunctiva is white and quiet and the hemorrhage is limited by the corneal limbus.*

Chapter 5

CORNEA

KAMBIZ NEGAHBAN

CORNEAL INFECTIONS

HISTORY

- Sudden onset of pain, copious yellow-green discharge from one eye
- History of contact lens wear, previous corneal or systemic illness, recent swimming with contact lenses, trauma or corneal foreign body, corneal transplant
- Symptoms: red eye, decreased vision, ocular pain, yellowish discharge

FINDINGS ON EXAMINATION

COMMON

- Usually acute and unilateral
- Red, injected conjunctiva
- Purulent discharge (Fig. 5-1)
- Tearing
- Light sensitivity
- Focal white infiltrate and ulcer in the corneal stroma with corneal stromal loss (Figs. 5-1 and 5-2)
- Surrounding corneal edema

- Descemet's membrane folds: appear as linear streaks on the posterior surface of the cornea if examined with a slit lamp
- Anterior chamber cells (best examined on the slit lamp with a 1-mm, narrow slit beam with bright illumination)

LESS COMMON

- Layering of white blood cells in anterior chamber (hypopyon) (Fig. 5-1)
- Previous foreign bodies or rust ring
- Corneal thinning and perforation: refer *urgently to an ophthalmologist*
- Leakage of aqueous fluid
- Posterior synechiae: adhesions between the iris and the anterior lens capsule, most commonly at the pupillary border

UNCOMMON

Should prompt further investigation for other causes.

- Blood in the anterior chamber (hyphema)
- Subconjunctival hemorrhage

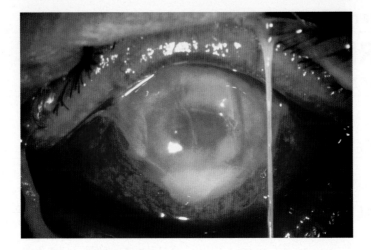

Figure 5-1 *Severe corneal infection with copious purulent discharge, white fluffy corneal infiltrates, and a layer of white blood cells in the anterior chamber (hypopyon). The infiltrate obscures the view of the underlying iris details.*

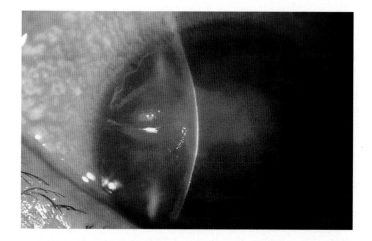

Figure 5-2 *Dense central stromal infiltrate caused by a corneal infection by* Acanthamoeba.

EXAMINATION OUTLINE

- Instill a drop of proparacaine (topical anesthetic) if patient is unable to open eye to cooperate because of pain. *Check corneal sensitivity first!*
- Rough check of visual acuity.
- External examination: carefully look for any skin rashes or vesicles that might suggest herpes simplex virus or varicella zoster infection (See also, section "Herpetic Infection"); note any eyelid swelling, scar, or fresh evidence of trauma to the periocular region
- Slit lamp examination: have patient remove his or her contact lenses if not already done
- Examine the cornea for focal white infiltrate or ulcer; an ulcer exists if there is also stromal loss with an overlying epithelial defect that stains with fluorescein; note if there are any satellite lesions, which would suggest a fungal infection; examine the location (central or peripheral) and size of the ulcer with the slit beam or a regular ruler if a slit lamp is not available
- Instill a drop of fluorescein in eye or touch conjunctival surface with a fluorescein strip moistened with sterile saline or sterile water and examine with cobalt blue light; use a Woods lamp or the cobalt blue filter of a direct ophthalmoscope if a slit lamp is not immediately available; look for highlighted epithelial defects
- Perform a Seidel test to detect aqueous leak and perforation
- Examine the inferior anterior chamber carefully to rule out a hypopyon (layering of white blood cells due to gravity in the anterior chamber)

TREATMENT

- Discontinue contact lens wear.
- Ulcers and infiltrates are generally treated as bacterial until laboratory studies reveal the causative organism or until a therapeutic trial is unsuccessful

SMALL PERIPHERAL ULCERS   If an ophthalmologist cannot be consulted urgently, small non-staining peripheral infiltrate in a noncontact lens wearer can be treated empirically with regular strength broad-spectrum antibiotics without prior scraping for cultures. Consider using broad-spectrum topical antibiotic (ofloxacin or ciprofloxacin) drops q 2 to 6 hours.

VISION THREATENING ULCERS   Large (greater than 1.5 mm in diameter) and central ulcers should be referred to an ophthalmologist *immediately* for work up, culturing, and fortified antibiotic drops.

- If corneal thinning is suspected, a fox shield *without* a patch should protect the eye until patient is seen by an ophthalmologist
- Consider admission to hospital if the patient is unable to self-administer the antibiotics, high likelihood of noncompliance, or large corneal ulcer

FOLLOW UP

- Patient should be followed up daily by an ophthalmologist to have accurate measurements of the size of the infiltrate and ulcer

- Always refer management of a large corneal ulcer to an ophthalmologist on an urgent basis, since a corneal transplant or patch graft might be considered if there is an impending or completed corneal perforation

PEARLS

- *Never* patch an infected eye.
- Acanthamoeba should be suspected in a contact lens wearer with history of poor lens hygiene or recent swimming. Pain is usually out of proportion to the extent of clinical findings.
- Suspect a sterile noninfectious ulcer if the eye is white and comfortable.
- Emphasize absolute discontinuation of contact lens wear to patients.
- If the ulcer was caused by trauma with organic material (sticks, leaves, etc.), be wary of fungal or gram-negative *(Bacillus)* organisms.

ICD-9 CODES

370.0	Corneal ulcer, unspecified
370.01	Corneal ulcer, marginal
370.03	Corneal ulcer, central
370.04	Corneal ulcer, hypopyon
370.05	Fungal ulcer

CONTACT LENS KERATITIS AND INFECTION

HISTORY

TYPE OF COMPLAINT   Mild pain, severe discomfort, itching, discharge, photophobia, decreased vision.

TYPE OF CONTACT LENS USED   Hard, soft, toric, bifocal, disposable, or extended wear.

DURATION   Age of the contact lenses, time of last fitting and used, overnight wear.

MAINTENANCE   Type of solution used with any recent changes in habits or solution, enzymatic tablet use, and history of allergy to preservatives, mainly thimerosal, benzalkonium chloride, or chlorohexidine.

FINDINGS ON EXAMINATION

DEPENDENT ON THE ETIOLOGY

Corneal Ulcer and Infiltrate

- Central and peripheral opacity with epithelial erosion and deeper tissue loss
- May have surrounding corneal edema causing haziness obscuring the underlying iris details

Corneal Epithelial Problems

- Common, with wide variation in appearances including epithelial thickening, punctate epithelial erosions (PEE), and corneal abrasions to pseudodendrites
- Can be secondary to traumatic and toxic reaction to the contact lenses
- Fluorescein staining of mainly central, 3 and 9 o'clock positions of the cornea

Toxicity and Hypersensitivity to Cleaning Solutions

- Chronic low-grade red eye with contact lens use or a recent change in contact lens solution
- Common with older type of cleaning agents
- Signs: diffuse pattern of PEE, conjunctival injection especially around the limbus, subepithelial infiltrates (Fig. 5-3), bulbar and palpebral conjunctival follicles (raised focal lymphoid nodules with accessory vascularization)

Giant Papillary Conjunctivitis (GPC)

- Large superior tarsal papillae (more than 0.3 mm in size) (Fig. 5-4), thickening and hyperemia of the superior tarsus
- More common in soft contact lens users than hard contact lens wearers
- Symptoms: red eye, itching, excessive mucoid discharge, blurred vision from mucous coating on contact lens, decreased contact lens wearing time

Tight Contact Lens Syndrome

- Punctate epithelial erosions, lack of movement of contact lens with blinking, conjunctival injection, imprint of the contact lens on the cornea, anterior chamber reaction with occasional hypopyon (layering of white blood cells inferiorly in the anterior chamber), limbal flush
- History of recent contact lens fitting or new contact lenses within the past 1 to 2 days

Pseudosuperior Limbic Keratoconjunctivitis

- Superior bulbar conjunctival injection and fluorescein staining
- Occasional subepithelial haze and infiltrates

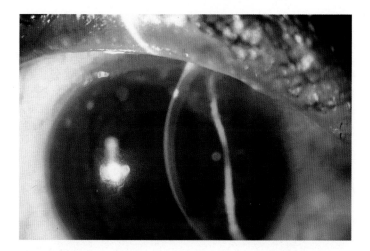

Figure 5-3 *Discrete, round superficial subepithelial infiltrates associated with contact lens wear. Large and central infiltrates should be managed by an ophthalmologist.*

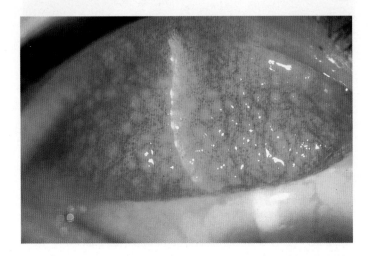

Figure 5-4 *Multiple giant papillae in a contact lens wearer. Chronic irritation of the tarsal conjunctiva results in inflammation and dilation and scarring of the pinpoint blood vessels resulting in these bumps.*

EXAMINATION OUTLINE

- Check rough visual acuity with contact lenses or glasses; if patient has no glasses, use the pinhole of the occluder
- If the patient still has the contact lens on, check the movement of the contact lens and any deposits or defects at the slit lamp
- Ask the patient to remove the contact lens; if unable to do so secondary to pain, may instill one drop of proparacaine or other topical anesthetic to open the eye to cooperate
- Examine contact lenses for tears or crusted deposits
- Check the reactivity of pupil with penlight
- Slit lamp examination with attention given to bulbar and palpebral conjunctiva to look for any papillae or follicles, corneal surface to rule out a corneal ulcer, and anterior chamber for reaction
- Evert the upper eyelids to look for giant papillae
- Instill a drop of fluorescein dye or touch conjunctival surface with moistened fluorescein strip and examine with cobalt blue light; note the location and staining of the conjunctiva and corneal surface
- Dilate the pupils after checking for narrow angles if history and presentation is atypical

TREATMENT

- *Remove and discontinue contact lens wear*
- Contact lens wearers with pain or redness should have thorough ophthalmological examination as soon as possible
- If an infectious etiology is suspected, patient needs to have a thorough examination by an ophthalmologist on an urgent basis to rule out a corneal ulcer

- If there is no timely access to an ophthalmologist: obtain smears and cultures of the ulcer with a small spatula; start broad-spectrum topical antibiotics with gram negative coverage such as a fluoroquinolone (e.g., ofloxacin or ciprofloxacin) 6 to 8 times per day and a cycloplegic drop (scopolamine 0.25% BID); refer promptly to an ophthalmologist
- Never patch an infected eye
- Treatment for noninfectious etiologies should be initiated by an ophthalmologist

FOLLOW UP

- If infectious, patients are reevaluated daily
- If noninfectious, reevaluate in several days
- Refer to an ophthalmologist on an urgent basis for large or central ulcers or decreased vision

PEARLS

- Contact lens wearers have relative corneal anesthesia and are more prone to infections.
- Overnight contact lens wear increases the risk of corneal infection tenfold over patients who wear them daily.
- Discontinuing contact lens wear is important, especially in young adults, who are more likely to be noncompliant secondary to social issues.

ICD-9 CODES

371.82   Corneal disorder secondary to contact lens
918.1   Corneal abrasion

HERPETIC KERATITIS

HISTORY

SIGNS AND SYMPTOMS Red eye, pain, photophobia, decreased vision, and vesicular/erythematous skin rash.

LATERALITY Ninety percent are unilateral. Suspect atopy or immunosuppression in bilateral cases.

DURATION: Acute or chronic.

MEDICAL HISTORY History of contact lens wear or corneal abrasion; immune state, recent use of systemic or topical steroids; previous nasal, oral, or genital sores; recent stress (fever, flu, emotional or physical exhaustion, sunburn, or substantial ultraviolet exposure).

FINDINGS ON EXAMINATION

- Red, injected conjunctiva
- Swollen eyelids
- Tearing
- Light sensitivity (if associated with iritis or epithelial defect)

SKIN SIGNS Clear vesicles with occasional crusting, and erythematous base.

- Conjunctivitis: red, hyperemic conjunctiva
- Keratitis: can involve all layers of the cornea, with corneal epithelial disease being the most common

Epithelial Dendrites

- Herpes simplex virus (HSV): a striking branching lesion with terminal bulbs at the end of each branch
- Varicella zoster virus (VZV): thin, wavy epithelial lesion similar to tangled spaghetti (Fig. 5-5A)

Neurotrophic (Sterile) Ulcer An opacity involving epithelial defect, stromal loss, and/or inflammation with smooth rolled edges usually located in the interpalpebral zone.

Corneal Stromal Disease Disk-shaped area of infiltrated stromal edema with or without an intact epithelium. Corneal stromal scars secondary to old infections may be present.

Iritis Cells in the anterior chamber, layer of white blood cells (hypopyon).

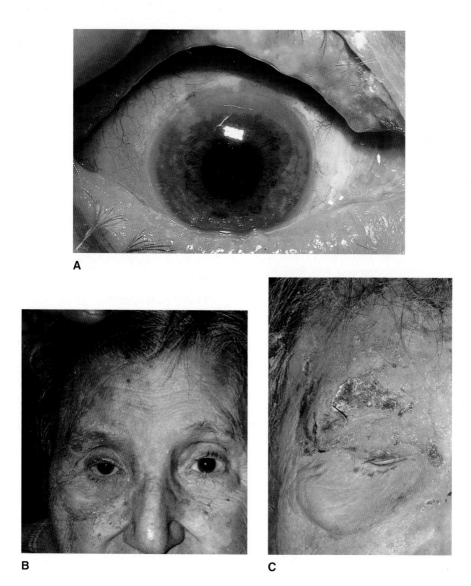

Figure 5-5 *A – C are from the same patient.*
A. Multiple epithelial dendritic lesions on the cornea of this patient with shingles. These are highlighted with the use of fluorescein dye.
B. Stereotypic skin rash of zoster affecting the right V1 distribution in the patient with the corneal findings in A. C. The rash resolves in the patient, leaving necrosis of the skin and a thick eschar.

EXAMINATION OUTLINE

- Rough check of visual acuity.
- Instill a drop of proparacaine or any topical anesthetic if the patient is unable to open eye to cooperate; *check corneal sensation before instilling topical anesthetic if possible*
- Note the relative distribution of skin vesicles if any (Fig. 5-5B and C)
- Check reactivity of pupils with penlight
- Slit lamp examination with attention given to determine the layer of cornea involved
- Instill a drop of fluorescein dye or touch conjunctival surface with moistened fluorescein strip and examine with cobalt blue light. Check for highlighted epithelial defects, PEE, or dendrites (Fig. 5-6)
- If available, counterstain with Rose Bengal or lissamine green
- Dilate pupil; any suspected herpetic infection should have a full dilated examination to rule out posterior pole findings

TREATMENT

CORNEAL EPITHELIAL DISEASE

- HSV: initiate treatment with trifluorothymidine 1% drops (Viroptic) 9 times per day or vidarabine 3% ointment (Vira-A) 5 times per day in the affected eye
- VZV: acyclovir 800 mg po 5 times per day
- Treatment for other ocular manifestations of HSV or VZV should generally be initiated by an experienced ophthalmologist
- If photophobia is present, may add a cycloplegic agent (e.g., scopolamine 0.25% TID) to reduce iris spasm and improve comfort
- If the area of involvement is extensive, consider gentle debridement of the infected epithelium as an adjunct to the antiviral agents; use a sterile, cotton-tip applicator or semisharp instrument under topical proparacaine anesthesia

FOLLOW UP

Patients should be referred to an ophthalmologist within 24 hours to ensure correct diagnosis and treatment. They are then reexamined every 2 to 5 days to evaluate clinical response to treatment.

PEARLS

Dendrites can be seen in many other conditions besides herpes simplex or zoster keratitis.

- Cytomegalovirus
- Adenovirus
- Contact lens or acanthamoeba keratitis pseudodendrites

A good and detailed history is very important in evaluating any dendritic corneal lesions. Patient should be told to avoid close contact with others. The fluid in the skin vesicles contains active infective viral particles.

ICD-9 CODES

053.20	VZV, dermatitis
053.21	VZV, keratoconjunctivitis
054.42	HSV, dendritic
054.43	HSV, disciform
054.49	HSV, other

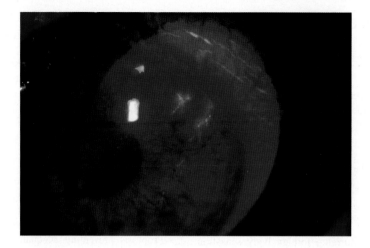

Figure 5-6 *Classic branching herpes simplex dendrite stained with fluorescein dye.*

EXPOSURE KERATOPATHY

HISTORY

- Exposure keratopathy is damage to the ocular surface secondary to drying because of poor or incomplete lid closure
- Inquire about history of previous Bell's palsy, sleep apnea, eyelid surgery, or thyroid eye disease
- History of autoimmune disease or chemical injury to the eyes

NOCTURNAL LAGOPHTHALMOS Inquire if any family members have seen the patient sleeping with eyes slightly open.

SYMPTOMS Burning, foreign body sensation ("sand or gritty feeling in the eyes"), tearing, redness, usually worse in the morning, may wake up at night with sharp pain in the eye.

LATERALITY Exposure keratopathy secondary to Grave's disease or eyelid surgery is usually bilateral.

FINDINGS ON EXAMINATION

- Incomplete blink or lagophthalmos
- Punctate epithelial erosions (PEE) that appear as fine, slightly depressed stippling caused by altered or desquamated superficial epithelium on the lower third of the cornea or as a horizontal band in the region of the palpebral fissure

OTHER SIGNS

- Red, injected conjunctiva
- Irregular epithelium (Fig. 5-7A)
- Corneal ulcer: an opacity with epithelial defect, stromal loss, or areas of inflammation
- Abnormal lid contour and closure (Fig. 5-7B)
- Proptosis preventing adequate lid closures, such as with thyroid eye disease
- Poor Bell's reflex (Table 5-1)

TABLE 5-1 TESTING FOR BELL'S REFLEX

- The eyes normally roll upwards with eyelid closure.
- Ask the patient to close his or her eyes forcefully.
- The examiner should pull the eyelids apart and see if the globe is rotated upward.
- A positive Bell's reflex is when the globe can be seen to be rotated upward.
- A negative Bell's reflex is when the globe remains positioned straight ahead.

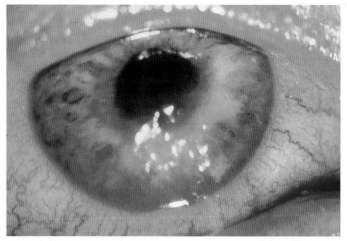

A

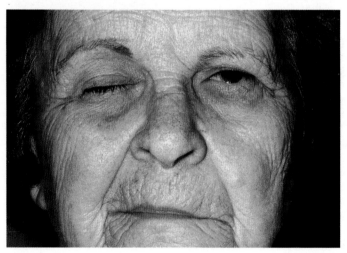

B

Figure 5-7 *A and B are from the same patient. **A.** Irregular epithelium in the interpalpebral fissue corresponding to the area exposed when the lids are closed. **B.** On closure of the eyelids, the right eye closes completely, but the left cornea remains exposed.*

EXAMINATION OUTLINE

- Check visual acuity
- Instill a drop of proparacaine or topical anesthetic if patient is unable to open eye to cooperate because of pain
- Evaluate eyelid closure: check for lagophthalmos by asking the patient to gently close his or her eyes as if sleeping, and measure amount of incomplete closure of the eyelids; assess Bell's reflex; if present, the area of drying may be covered by lower lid when awake; check for any eyelid distortion or scarring from previous trauma
- Slit lamp examination
- Instill a drop of fluorescein dye or touch conjunctival surface with moistened fluorescein strip and examine with cobalt blue light; this can be done with a direct handheld ophthalmoscope if no slit lamp is immediately available; Rose Bengal or lissamine green can also highlight affected areas
- Look for highlighted epithelial defects and punctate staining; check carefully for any areas of possible corneal ulcer (see "Findings on Examination")

TREATMENT

- Frequent topical artificial tears and ointments q 1 to 6 hours depending on the amount of staining and degree of exposure
- Increase ambient air humidity by having a humidifier at home
- Consider taping or patching the eyelid closed at night to maintain eyelids in the closed position; this is usually a temporary measure until definitive surgery can be done to correct eyelid position.

- In addition to above therapy, in severely affected individuals moist chamber goggles or plastic wrap over the eyes help prevent moisture evaporation
- Treatment of the underlying condition
- Definitive treatment may be partial surgical closure of the eyelids

FOLLOW UP

- If there is no corneal ulcer, patient is reexamined in few weeks to months to evaluate therapy success; patient can be referred to an ophthalmologist in few weeks for follow up
- If there is evidence of corneal ulcer or infiltrate, patient should be seen by an ophthalmologist on an urgent basis

PEARLS

- Family members and spouse are important in eliciting history of nocturnal lagophthalmos.

- If patient appears obese or has history of sleep apnea, he or she may have floppy eyelid syndrome, where the upper eyelids are easily everted during sleep and may rub on the pillow or sheets.

- Surgical intervention in treating exposure keratopathy refractory to noninvasive interventions is very successful and sight saving in extreme cases.

ICD-9 CODES

370.2	Lagophthalmos, unspecified
370.34	Exposure keratoconjunctivitis
374.21	Lagophthalmos, paralytic
374.22	Lagophthalmos, mechanical

DRY EYES (KERATOCONJUNCTIVITIS SICCA)

HISTORY (SEE TABLE 5-2)

DURATION AND LATERALITY Usually chronic and bilateral.

MEDICATION HISTORY Anticholinergics or antihistamines, oral contraceptives, beta blockers, phenothiazines, and atropine.

COLLAGEN VASCULAR DISEASES Sjögren's syndrome, rheumatoid arthritis, systemic lupus erythematosus, and Wegener's granulomatosis.

LOW-HUMIDITY ENVIRONMENTS Airplanes, air-conditioned rooms, or desert climate.

HISTORY Contact lens wear or chemical injury to the eyes. Radiation treatment to the head and neck area.

EXACERBATING FACTORS Smoke, wind, heat, low humidity, and alcohol consumption.

LACRIMAL INFILTRATION Sarcoidosis of lymphoma.

SYMPTOMS RELATED TO DRY EYES

- Burning or foreign body sensation (sandy, gritty sensation)
- Red eyes
- Blurred vision secondary to disruption of the tear film
- Photophobia (light sensitivity)

TABLE 5-2 **MAJOR CAUSES OF KERATOCONJUNCTIVITIS SICCA**

- Increased evaporation
  - Increased eyelid fissure height (thyroid eye disease, previous blepharoplasty)
  - Decreased blink (Parkinson's syndrome)
  - Incomplete blink (lagophthalmos, cicatricial lid changes)
- Decreased tear production
  - Sjögren's syndrome
  - Use of anticholinergic agents
- Unstable tear film
  - Blepharitis
  - Meibomitis
  - Irregular corneal epithelial surface

FINDINGS ON EXAMINATION

- Red, injected conjunctiva worse as the day progresses
- Mild to moderate thickening of the lid margins with dilated telangiectatic vessels
- Decreased tear lake with clumps of mucus in tears (Fig. 5-8)
- Oily discharge from meibomian gland orifices
- Oil or excessive mucus or debris in the tear film
- Lagophthalmos (incomplete closure of the eyelids); see section "Exposure Keratopathy" for testing procedure to detect lagophthalmos
- Staining of cornea and conjunctiva in the interpalpebral fissure with Rose Bengal or lissamine green (Fig. 5-9)
- Decreased tear break-up time (see section "Examination Outline")

UNCOMMON

Should prompt further investigation for other causes.

- Anterior chamber inflammation
- Stromal infiltrate or ulcer
- Purulent discharge

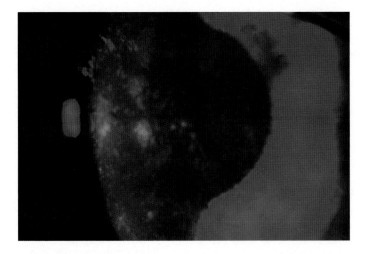

Figure 5-8 *Patchy staining of mucus on the cornea in a patient with dry eyes. A normal patient has a uniform tear film with no staining.*

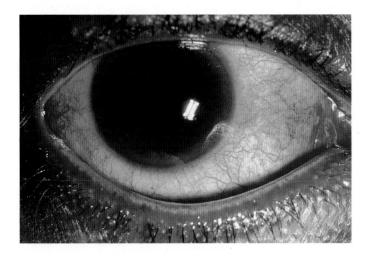

Figure 5-9 *Rose Bengal instilled into the eye highlights areas of damaged conjunctival epithelium. The interpalpebral band of staining is typical of dry eyes.*

TABLE 5-3 ROSACEA

Idiopathic condition characterized by
- Recurrent papules
- Pustules
- Unpredictable flushing episodes
- Rhinophyma—thickening of the skin and connective tissue of the nose

Sometimes associated with the consumption of
- Alcohol, coffee, spicy foods

EXAMINATION OUTLINE

- Check visual acuity
- Instill a drop of proparacaine (topical anesthetic) if patient is unable to open eye to cooperate because of pain

EXTERNAL EXAMINATION Examine the skin for any changes that might suggest collagen vascular diseases or rosacea (Table 5-3). Check for lagophthalmos by asking the patient to close his or her eyes gently as if sleeping, and check to see if the upper eyelids and the lower eyelids are in complete apposition. Note any possible enlargement of the lacrimal glands (superotemporal part of the eyes) to suggest infiltrative process (e.g., sarcoidosis).

- Slit lamp examination
- Examine the eyelid margins carefully to identify any thickening, telangiectatic vessels, or oily discharge that would suggest a diagnosis of blepharitis (inflammation of the eyelids).
- Observe the tear film to detect oil, debris, or make-up

- Instill a drop of fluorescein dye or touch conjunctival surface with moistened fluorescein strip and examine with cobalt blue light; this can be done with the cobalt blue feature of a direct ophthalmoscope if a slit lamp is not available
- Look for highlighted epithelial defects or PEE across the cornea, usually in the interpalpebral region
- Measure tear break-up time; this is performed by asking the patient to blink once only and the examiner simultaneously counting and examining the corneal surface to detect a tear film defect by using fluorescein stain (Table 5-4)
- Dilate pupil if presentation is atypical with significant visual loss

TABLE 5-4 TEAR BREAK-UP TIME

1–5 sec	Rapid break up
5–10 sec	Borderline
Greater than 10 sec	Normal

TREATMENT

Treat underlying cause. If the patient has evidence of blepharitis, may initiate therapy by:

- Scrubbing the eyelid margins with mild shampoo (e.g., Johnson's baby shampoo) twice a day on a cotton-tipped applicator or a warm washcloth
- Warm compresses for 10 to 15 min BID

MILD   Initiate therapy with artificial tears QID (e.g., Refresh Tears, Genteal, HypoTears, Tears Naturale II).

MODERATE   If the previous therapy is not successful, consider increasing frequency of artificial tear application to every 1 to 2 h with *preservative-free* artificial tears (e.g., Refresh Plus, Bion Tears, Celluvisc) and adding a lubricating ointment at bedtime (e.g., Lacrilube). Decrease evaporative loss with increased humidity or moist chambers.

SEVERE   If moderate therapy is not successful, refer to an ophthalmologist in a few weeks to consider punctal occlusion with collagen or silicone plugs or surgical partial closure of the eyelid.

FOLLOW UP

- Patient may be followed up in few days to weeks depending on the severity of the drying changes and symptoms
- If patient's symptoms are not relieved by moderate therapy, refer to an ophthalmologist in few weeks to consider punctal plugs

PEARLS

- Dry eye syndrome is a chronic and bilateral disease. Some patients, however, are seen with a recent onset in one eye only. It is one of the most common causes of chronic low-grade irritations of the eyes, particularly in the elderly population. It often causes more discomfort than the clinical signs would suggest.

- Always use preservative-free artificial tears if using them more frequently than every 4 h to prevent preservative toxicity.

- Refer to an internist or rheumatologist for further evaluation if the history suggests the presence of a previously undiagnosed collagen vascular disease.

- Discourage patients with significant dry eyes from contact lens wear. Contact lens wearers have a high rate of intolerance to contact lens wear.

ICD-9 CODES

370.33	Keratoconjunctivitis sicca, not specified as Sjögren's
373.00	Blepharitis
375.15	Tear film insufficient (dry eye)
710.2	Sjögren's syndrome

Chapter 6

UVEITIS

KENNETH C. CHERN

IRIDOCYCLITIS AND TRAUMATIC IRITIS

HISTORY

- Photophobia
- Redness
- Unilateral or bilateral disease
- Previous episodes
- History of trauma or eye infections

OCULAR FINDINGS

- Conjunctival injection
- Perilimbal flush
- Keratic precipitates (Fig. 6-1)
- Synechiae (anterior or posterior)
- Anterior chamber cell and flare
- Increase or decrease in intraocular pressure

SEVERE INFLAMMATION

- Fibrin in anterior chamber
- Hypopyon (Fig. 6-2)
- Fibrinoid membrane on lens capsule

EXAMINATION OUTLINE

- Check vision
- Slit lamp examination—use high magnification, small slit, and bright light to look for cells suspended in the aqueous humor
- Instill fluorescein to stain surface for dendritic disease or ulcers
- Check intraocular pressure
- Dilate pupil

WORK UP

In severe cases of inflammation or recurrent episodes, laboratory studies may be helpful in determining the cause. (See Table 6-1.)

- Angiotensin converting enzyme (ACE)
- Lysozyme
- HLA-B27
- Chest x-ray
- PPD and controls
- Lyme titers
- Antinuclear antibody levels
- Rheumatoid factor

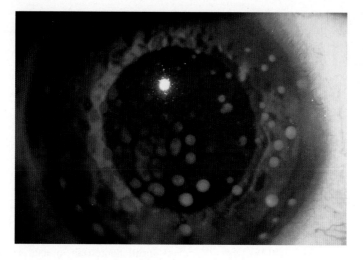

Figure 6-1 *Greyish-white deposits (keratic precipitates) on the endothelial surface in a patient with granulomatous anterior uveitis associated with sarcoidosis.*

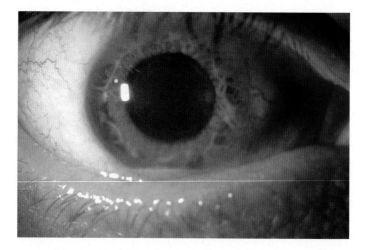

Figure 6-2 *Layering of white blood cells inferiorly in the anterior chamber (hypopyon) in a case of severe anterior uveitis associated with HLA-B27.*

TABLE 6-1 COMMON CAUSES OF IRIDOCYCLITIS

Inflammatory conditions
- HLA-B27 associated
- Sarcoidosis
- Juvenile rheumatoid arthritis

Infections
- Herpes simplex
- Varicella zoster
- Syphilis
- Toxoplasmosis
- Corneal infections

Trauma

Idiopathic

TREATMENT

- Topical steroid drops (prednisolone 1%)
- Subconjunctival or oral steroids for severe inflammation
- Cycloplegics—improves ocular comfort, dilates pupil
- Treat elevated IOP with antihypertensive drops

FOLLOW UP

See ophthalmologist within a week, more urgently with severe inflammation.

PEARLS

- As the inflammation resolves, the keratic precipitates become smaller and more pigmented; they may not disappear completely.

- If an infection by bacteria or virus is suspected, do not begin steroid therapy. Refer urgently to an ophthalmologist.

ICD-9 CODES

364.00	Acute/subacute iridocyclitis
364.02	Recurrent iridocyclitis
364.05	Hypopyon
364.10	Chronic iridocyclitis

SCLERITIS

HISTORY

- Deep, boring pain—globe tender to touch
- Redness
- History of rheumatologic or collagen–vascular diseases

OCULAR FINDINGS

- Conjunctival and deep scleral injection (Fig. 6-3)
- Swollen scleral nodules
- Scleral thinning
- Necrotic and avascular areas of sclera (Fig. 6-4)

EXAMINATION OUTLINE

- Check vision
- Examination of the sclera in natural light looking for a deep red or purple hue
- Slit lamp examination
- Dilate pupil

WORK UP

In severe cases of scleritis, patients may have an underlying systemic autoimmune disease such as rheumatoid arthritis, systemic lupus erythematosis, Wegener's granulomatosis, and polyarteritis nodosa. Patients should be referred to their internist for examination and blood work.

TREATMENT

- Oral nonsteroidal anti-inflammatory medications (e.g., indomethacin)
- Systemic steroids
- Immunosuppression for severe necrotizing cases or recalcitrant disease

FOLLOW UP

See ophthalmologist within a week.

PEARLS

- The most common systemic disease associated with scleritis is rheumatoid arthritis.

- Scleritis can also occur secondary to infections from organisms such as *Nocardia, Acanthamoeba,* and *Pseudomonas.*

ICD-9 CODES

379.00   Scleritis

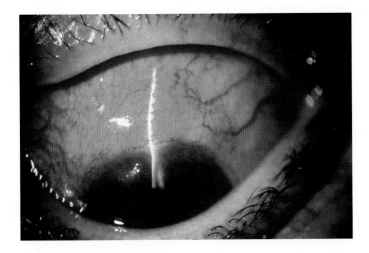

Figure 6-3 *Diffuse conjunctival and scleral inflammation superiorly on this eye. Note the pinkish-yellow swelling of the sclera indicated by the contour of the thin slit beam.*

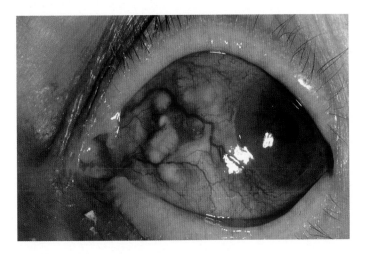

Figure 6-4 *Severe necrotizing scleritis with loss of scleral tissue in this rheumatoid arthritis patient. The brownish hue visible at the base of the ulcer is the underlying choroid.*

ENDOPHTHALMITIS

HISTORY

- Gradual or sudden onset of pain, decreased vision, ocular redness
- History of recent intraocular surgery
- Penetrating ocular trauma

OCULAR FINDINGS

- Decreased vision, can be mild or dramatic
- Conjunctival injection
- Anterior chamber inflammation and hypopyon (Figs. 6-5 and 6-6)
- Whitish deposits on or behind the lens
- Obscured view of the optic nerve and retinal details secondary to vitreous inflammation

WORK UP

- Vitreous tap and cultures by ophthalmologist (See Table 6-2.)
- B-scan ultrasound to examine extent of inflammation

TREATMENT

- Hourly topical fortified broad-spectrum antibiotics: cefazolin or vancomycin, gentamicin or tobramycin
- Subconjunctival antibiotic injections
- Vitrectomy surgery and intravitreal antibiotic injections

FOLLOW UP

- Urgent referral to an ophthalmologist, especially in cases of ocular trauma

PEARLS

Postoperative endophthalmitis following cataract surgery can occur weeks to years after the initial surgery.

ICD-9 CODES

360.01   Acute endophthalmitis
360.03   Chronic endophthalmitis

CPT CODES

65810   Vitreous biopsy
67028   Intravitreal injection

TABLE 6-2 COMMON ORGANISMS CAUSING ENDOPHTHALMITIS

Traumatic	*Bacillus, Staphylococcus, Streptococcus*
Post-operative	
Acute	*Staphylococcus, Streptococcus*
Chronic	*Propionibacterium acnes, Staphylococcus epidermidus, Streptococcus,* fungi
Endogeneous	Fungi, gram-negative organisms

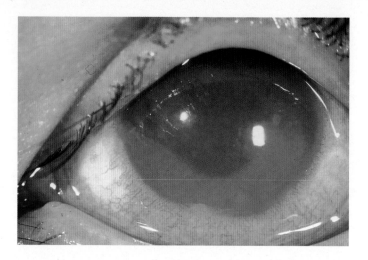

Figure 6-5 *Diffuse anterior segment inflammation with obscuration of iris details secondary to white blood cells and fibrin within the anterior chamber. The hypopyon and diffuse conjunctival injections are also suggestive of endophthalmitis.*

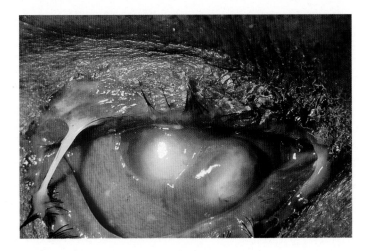

Figure 6-6 *Traumatic injury with rupture of the globe and extensive ocular inflammation and infection involving the vitreous, anterior chamber, and rupture site. The lens capsule has also been damaged allowing hydration and whitening of the lens.*

Chapter 7

LENS

KENNETH C. CHERN

CATARACT FORMATION

DEFINITION A cataract is any opacification (focal or diffuse) of the lens. It may or may not affect vision (Table 7-1)

HISTORY

- Decreased vision, blurring or haziness to vision
- Glare or starbursts around lights
- Difficulty seeing in dim light or darkness
- Metabolic disorders such as diabetes mellitus, Wilson's disease
- History of phenothiazine or corticosteroid use, acute angle closure glaucoma

FINDINGS

- Diffuse yellow-brown discoloration of the lens (nuclear sclerosis) (Fig. 7-1)
- Focal lenticular opacities can be opaque wedges (cortical wedges) (Fig. 7-2), Y-shaped opacities, or focal spots (Fig. 7-3)
- Complete opacification and whitening of cataract (mature cataract) (Fig. 7-4)

OCULAR EXAMINATION

- Vision, with glare source if indicated
- Check pupils; cataracts normally do not cause an afferent pupillary defect
- Dilate pupil
- Slit lamp exam
- If no view of fundus, obtain B-scan ultrasound to investigate posterior segment

TREATMENT

Refer to ophthalmologist for evaluation and possible cataract surgery (Fig. 7-5)

PEARLS

- Senile cataracts are often symmetric bilaterally.
- Asymmetric cataracts should warrant further evaluation for a cause.

ICD-9 CODES

366.14 Cataract, posterior subcapsular
366.15 Cataract, senile cortical
366.16 Cataract, nuclear sclerosis

TABLE 7-1 COMMON CAUSES FOR CATARACTS

Type	Common Cause
Polar	Congenital
Nuclear sclerosis (see Fig. 7-1)	Aging
Cortical spokes (see Fig. 7-2)	Aging
Posterior subcapsular (Fig. 7-6)	Steroid use Previous intraocular surgery Ocular inflammation
Snowflake and focal opacities (see Fig. 7-3)	Diabetes High intraocular pressure and glaucoma
Focal opacities	Trauma
Mature white cataract (see Fig. 7-4)	Trauma Aging
Capsular deposits (Fig. 7-7)	Drugs (phenothiazines, in particular) Elevated serum iron or copper levels

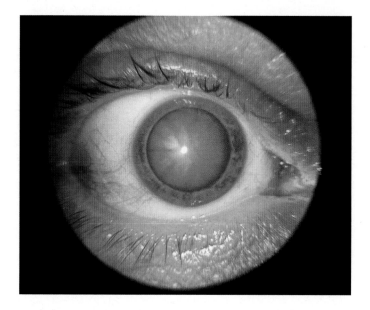

Figure 7-1 *A nuclear sclerotic cataract causes gradual obscuration of vision like looking through murky water. On examination, the lens has a brownish-yellow discoloration.*

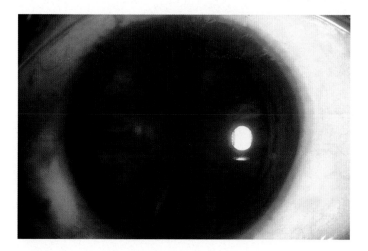

Figure 7-2 *The radial spoke-like cortical opacities of the lens are very symptomatic, since they scatter light and increase glare. This is particularly troublesome at night because headlights and street lights will appear as starbursts.*

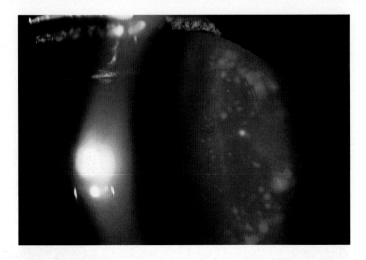

Figure 7-3 *Focal lenticular opacities caused by diabetes. Most of these opacities are small enough that they do not affect vision.*

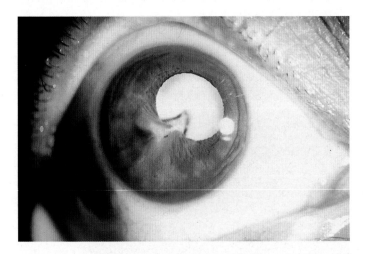

Figure 7-4 *Traumatic cataract with complete whitening of the lens. The visual acuity in this patient was light perception.*

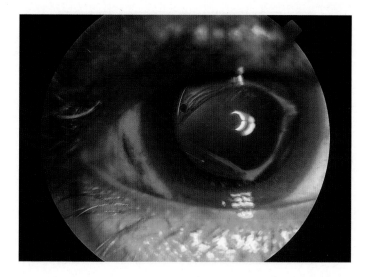

Figure 7-5 *Following cataract surgery, an artificial lens is placed to provide focusing power for the eye. In many cases, the lens is difficult to see except for the two light reflexes from the anterior and posterior lens surfaces. The diamond-shaped whitish outline is the fibrotic remnant of the lens capsule.*

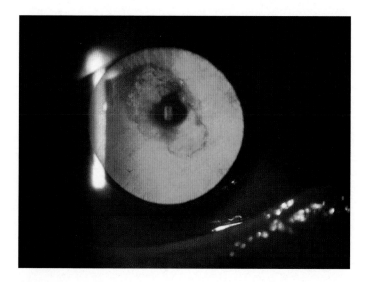

Figure 7-6 *A posterior subcapsular cataract appears as a plaque stuck on the posterior surface of the lens. These cataracts cause glare and interfere with reading.*

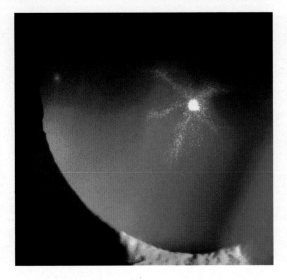

Figure 7-7 *Whitish stellate deposits in the anterior lens capsule are common in patients who are on chronic phenothiazine therapy.*

Chapter 8

GLAUCOMA

ROHIT KRISHNA

MICHAEL CASSELL

ANGLE CLOSURE GLAUCOMA

HISTORY

- Monocular pain
- Photophobia
- Red eye
- Blurred vision
- Rainbow-colored halos and starbursts around lights
- Nausea and vomiting
- May report previous attack in same or opposing eye

FINDINGS ON EXAMINATION

COMMON

- High intraocular pressure (usually higher than 40 mm Hg)
- Decreased visual acuity
- Red eye with congested blood vessels
- Mid-dilated, sluggish or nonreactive pupil, often irregularly shaped
- Corneal edema (cloudiness)
- Shallow anterior chamber

- Aqueous cell and flare on slit lamp examination

LESS COMMON

- Dense cataract
- Peripheral anterior synechiae—adhesions of the peripheral iris to the cornea
- Disk hemorrhage (Drance hemorrhage) (Fig. 8-1)

UNCOMMON

- Bilateral condition

EXAMINATION OUTLINE

- Check visual acuity
- Check reactivity of pupil with penlight
- Slit lamp examination
- Check for corneal edema
- Check anterior chamber depth and look for presence of aqueous cell and flare
- Examine iris for mid-dilation, irregular shape, and bowing forward (iris bombé)
- Examine lens for cataract
- Measure intraocular pressure by Schiotz tonometry, Tono-Pen, or Goldmann applanation tonometry

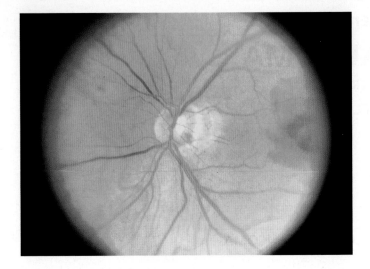

Figure 8-1 *Hemorrhage located at the 4 o'clock position of the optic nerve head. Such hemorrhages are associated with the development of a visual field defect corresponding to the arcuate bundle that courses over the optic nerve rim at the location of the hemorrhage.*

TREATMENT

- Lower intraocular pressure: (1) Acetazolamide 500 mg po (or IV if too nauseated for po medication); make sure patient does not have a sulfa allergy, blood dyscrasia, kidney disease, or other contraindication to thiazide diuretics; (2) instill timolol 0.5% if no contraindication to beta-blockers and brimonidine (Alphagan) or apraclonidine (Iopidine); (3) Oral glycerin or isosorbide
- Control pain and nausea, including use of narcotics if necessary
- Single dose pilocarpine 1% or 2% to pull iris away from angle
- Do not use dilating drops, which may worsen angle closure

FOLLOW UP

- Urgent ophthalmologic consultation upon diagnosis
- Definitive treatment usually laser or surgical iridotomy

PEARLS

- Bilateral angle closure is rare; consider other diagnoses.
- If intraocular pressure increases slowly, corneal edema may be mild or absent.
- If the pressure is less than 30 mm Hg, acute angle closure is unlikely. Consider other etiologies for pain.

ICD-9 CODES

365.22 Acute angle closure
365.23 Chronic angle closure

CPT CODE

66761 Laser peripheral iridectomy

HYPHEMA AND TRAUMATIC GLAUCOMA

HISTORY

- Blunt trauma
- Pain and photophobia in affected eye
- Decreased vision

FINDINGS ON EXAMINATION

COMMON

- Hyphema—blood in the anterior chamber (Fig 8-2; Table 8-1)

Associated ocular trauma:

- Corneal abrasion
- Iris sphincter tear
- Traumatic iritis

LESS COMMON

- Increased intraocular pressure (IOP), may be acute or late, secondary to obstruction of the trabecular meshwork by red cells or direct damage to intraocular structures
- Corneal blood staining, usually with large hyphemas, rebleeding, and elevated IOP

Associated ocular and orbital trauma:

- Lens subluxation
- Corneal or scleral rupture
- Intraocular foreign body
- Vitreous hemorrhage
- Retinal edema (commotio retinae) or detachment
- Orbital fracture

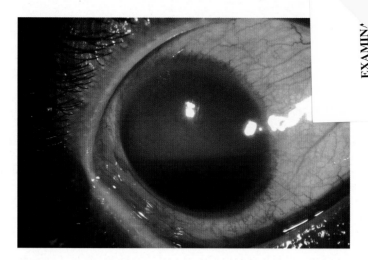

Figure 8-2 *Blunt trauma causing bleeding and layering of red blood cells in the anterior chamber (hyphema). Dispersed blood obscures the view of the iris details in this grade III hyphema.*

TABLE 8-1 **GRADING OF HYPHEMAS**

Grade I	Microhyphema: circulating red blood cells in anterior chamber without layering
Grade II	Layering less than one third of anterior chamber
Grade III	Layering one third to one half of anterior chamber
Grade IV	"Eight-ball" or total hyphema

...ION OUTLINE

. visual acuity
.eck reactivity of pupil with penlight
Check ocular motility
- Slit lamp examination
- Check cornea and sclera for rupture
- Examine anterior chamber for red blood cells and grade hyphema
- Check iris margin for sphincter tear
- Look for lens subluxation
- In absence of rupture, instill a drop of fluorescein dye or touch conjunctival surface with moistened fluorescein strip after instilling topical anesthetic, examine with cobalt blue light to look for epithelial defects
- Measure intraocular pressure by Schiotz tonometry, Tono-Pen, or Goldmann applanation tonometry
- Instill dilating drops and examine fundus
- Image orbits if corneal or scleral rupture or suspected orbital fracture

- If the patient is African American or has other risk factors for sickle cell disease and has not been previously tested, order a sickle cell prep

TREATMENT

- Metal or hard plastic shield to protect eye
- Limit activity to decrease incidence of rebleeding (usually within the first 3 to 7 days)
- Remain upright and elevate head of bed 45° while sleeping to allow the blood to settle inferiorly
- Cycloplegia for comfort (cyclopentolate 1% TID)
- Prednisolone acetate 1% QID to decrease inflammation
- If abrasion present, withhold prednisolone drops and treat abrasion with topical antibiotics until surface healed
- No aspirin or nonsteroidal anti-inflammatory medications

FOLLOW UP

REFER URGENTLY

- Corneal or scleral rupture
- Corneal staining
- Hyphema grade III or IV
- Intraocular pressure higher than 30 mm Hg
- Lens subluxation
- Vitreous hemorrhage, whitening of retina (retinal edema), or other fundus abnormality
- Unable to visualize fundus
- Monocular patient

CONSIDER ADMISSION

- Infant, toddler, or child requiring a controlled environment to limit activity
- Unreliable patient or caregiver

See ophthalmologist within 24 hours to assess degree of clearing, check intraocular pressure, and examine fundus.

ICD-9 CODE

364.41   Hyphema

BLEB-ASSOCIATED INFECTIONS

HISTORY

- Trabeculectomy (filtering procedure) for glaucoma in affected eye
- Pain
- Blurred vision
- Tearing
- Redness
- Discharge

FINDINGS ON EXAMINATION

COMMON (TABLE 8-2)

- Conjunctival injection
- Purulent discharge
- Milky-white, cloudy bleb (Fig. 8-3) with or without hypopyon (layering of purulent material within bleb)
- Corneal edema
- Cell and flare within anterior chamber
- Bleb leak demonstrated by positive Seidel test
- Intraocular pressure may be high, normal, or low

LESS COMMON

- Hypotony with flat anterior chamber
- Hypopyon (layering of white blood cells in anterior chamber)

EXAMINATION OUTLINE

- Check visual acuity
- Check reactivity of pupil with penlight
- Instill a drop of topical anesthetic
- Slit lamp examination
- Examine conjunctiva for injection
- Ask patient to look downward, lift eyelid with a cotton-tip swab, and examine the bleb; a healthy bleb is semitranslucent with little to no vasculature; an infected bleb is surrounded by injected blood vessels, has a cloudy or murky appearance, and may have a pseudohypopyon from layering of purulent material
- Check for corneal edema
- Examine anterior chamber for cell and flare
- Perform Seidel test

TABLE 8-2 GRADING OF BLEB INFECTIONS

Grade I	Blebitis without anterior chamber reaction; only the subconjunctival space is involved (bleb infection, injection)
Grade II	Blebitis with anterior chamber reaction; entire anterior segment is involved
Grade III	Bleb-related endophthalmitis; the anterior and posterior segment (retina and vitreous) are involved

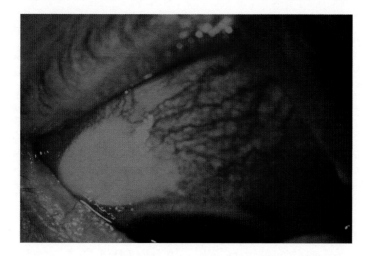

Figure 8-3 *Patient with previous trabeculectomy presenting with pain and decreased vision. Extensive conjunctival whitening of the glaucoma bleb from an infection.*

TREATMENT

- Grade I: fluoroquinolone drops [e.g., ofloxacin (Ocuflox), ciprofloxacin (Ciloxan), or levofloxacin (Quixin)] one drop every 1 to 2 h while awake
- Grade II: topical fortified cefazolin or vancomycin (25 mg/mL) plus fortified tobramycin (14 mg/mL) or amikacin (50 mg/mL) every hour
- Grade III: injection of intravitreal antibiotics with vitreous sampling or vitrectomy surgery by ophthalmologist, oral antibiotics, and topical fortified antibiotics; possible hospital admission

FOLLOW UP

- Grade I: contact ophthalmologist by telephone, see ophthalmologist within 24 h
- Grade II or III: urgent evaluation by ophthalmologist

ICD-9 CODES

360.01   Endophthalmitis, acute
360.03   Endophthalmitis, chronic
360.02   Panuveitis
360.19   Other endophthalmitis
372.03   Other mucopurulent conjunctivitis

PHACOLYTIC GLAUCOMA

HISTORY

- Monocular pain
- Red eye
- Blurred vision
- Haloes around lights

FINDINGS ON EXAMINATION

COMMON

- Markedly decreased visual acuity
- Conjunctival injection
- Corneal edema
- Granulomatous keratic precipitates (KP): fluffy brown or white deposits on the endothelial surface of the cornea
- Anterior chamber flare
- Mature white cataract (Fig. 8-4)
- Elevated intraocular pressure

EXAMINATION OUTLINE

- Check visual acuity
- Check reactivity of pupil with penlight
- Slit lamp examination
- Examine conjunctiva for injection
- Check for corneal edema
- Examine anterior chamber for flare
- Examine lens
- Check intraocular pressure with Goldmann applanation tonometer, Schiotz tonometer, or Tono-Pen

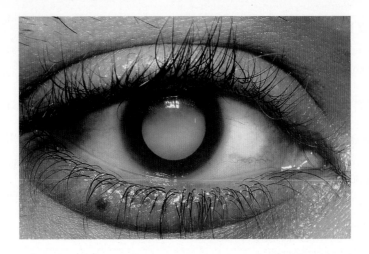

Figure 8-4 *White, mature cataract visible through the pupil. Patients can develop a small rent in the anterior capsule permitting leakage of lens proteins into the anterior chamber causing phacolytic glaucoma.*

TREATMENT

- Acetazolamide 500 mg po (or IV if too nauseated for po medication), then 500 mg BID or 250 mg QID; make sure patient does not have a sulfa allergy, blood dyscrasia, kidney disease, or other contraindication to thiazide diuretics
- Medical management of IOP with one or a combination of the following drops: timolol 0.5% if no contraindication to beta-blockers, bromonidine (Alphagan) or apraclonidine (Iopidine) BID
- Prednisolone 1%
- Cyclopentolate (Cyclogyl) 1% TID
- Definitive treatment is cataract extraction

FOLLOW UP

- Contact ophthalmologist by telephone, see ophthalmologist within 24 hours
- Urgent evaluation by ophthalmologist if IOP cannot be controlled (greater than 30 mm Hg) with medications

PEARLS

- Mechanism of elevated IOP is obstruction of the trabecular meshwork by lens proteins, which leak through the intact lens capsule of a hypermature cataract. Think "phaco-*leaky*" glaucoma.
- Does not occur in children.
- If no cataract is present, consider angle closure glaucoma.

ICD-9 CODES

365.59   Glaucoma associated with lens disorder
366.17   Mature cataract

NEOVASCULAR GLAUCOMA

HISTORY

- Monocular pain
- Red eye
- Poor vision
- Possible nausea and vomiting
- History of proliferative diabetic retinopathy, ocular vascular disease (central retinal artery or vein occlusion), sickle cell disease, collagen vascular disease, uveitis, retinal detachment, or intraocular tumor

FINDINGS

COMMON

- High intraocular pressure
- Decreased visual acuity (may be decreased due to diabetes or other conditions)
- Red eye with congested blood vessels
- Corneal edema (cloudiness)
- New abnormal blood vessels on the anterior surface of the iris (Fig. 8-5)

LESS COMMONHYPHEMA

- Hyphema

TREATMENT

- Decrease IOP using one or more of these pressure lowering drops: beta-blockers, brimonidine (Alphagan), latanoprost (Xalatan)

- Control pain and nausea, including use of narcotics if necessary
- Acetazolamide 500 mg po (or IV if too nauseated for oral medication); make sure patient does not have a sulfa allergy, blood dyscrasia, kidney disease, or other contraindication to thiazide diuretics

FOLLOW UP

Urgent ophthalmologic consultation upon diagnosis.

PEARLS

- Although medical management may temporarily decrease IOP, surgery is usually required for definitive pressure management.

- Treatment of underlying condition can cause vessels to regress, but glaucoma may persist.

ICD-9 CODES

364.42   Rubeosis iridis
365.63   Glaucoma associated with vascular disorders

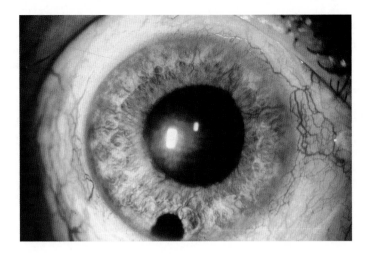

Figure 8-5 *Extensive neovascularization of the iris surface in a patient with a previous retinal detachment.*

PSEUDOEXFOLIATION SYNDROME

HISTORY

Usually asymptomatic.

EXAMINATION FINDINGS

- Pigment deposition on corneal endothelium
- "Moth-eaten" appearance of iris pupillary margin
- Target-shaped deposition of flaky white material on the lens and other ocular structures (Fig. 8-6)
- Intraocular pressure may be normal or elevated

TREATMENT

- Medical management of elevated IOP if present
- Decrease IOP using one or more of these pressure lowering drops: beta-blockers, brimonidine (Alphagan), latanoprost (Xalatan)
- Control pain and nausea, including use of narcotics if necessary

FOLLOW UP

Contact ophthalmologist by telephone if IOP elevated. Otherwise, routine evaluation by ophthalmologist as outpatient.

ICD-9 CODE

365.52   Pseudoexfoliative glaucoma

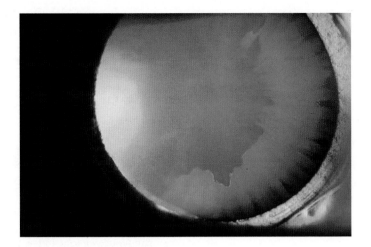

Figure 8-6 *Whitish pseudo-exfoliative material deposited on the anterior lens capsule. The central portion of the lens is free from the material.*

PIGMENTARY GLAUCOMA

HISTORY

Usually asymptomatic; may have episodes of blurred vision and haloes due to transient rises in IOP

FINDINGS ON EXAMINATION

- Intraocular pressure may be normal or elevated
- Krukenberg's spindle (vertical band of pigment on the corneal endothelium) (Fig. 8-7)
- Pigment in the anterior chamber after dilation
- Iris transillumination defects (loss of iris pigment)

TREATMENT

- Medical management of elevated IOP, if present
- Decrease IOP using one or more of these pressure lowering drops: beta-blockers, brimonidine (Alphagan), latanoprost (Xalatan)
- Control pain and nausea, including use of narcotics if necessary

FOLLOW UP

Evaluation by ophthalmologist as outpatient.

PEARLS

- Rare in patients younger than 50 years

- Highest pressures usually seen after heavy physical exertion, such as riding a bicycle, mountain climbing, or other strenuous workout (releases pigment)

ICD-9 CODE

365.13   Pigmentary glaucoma

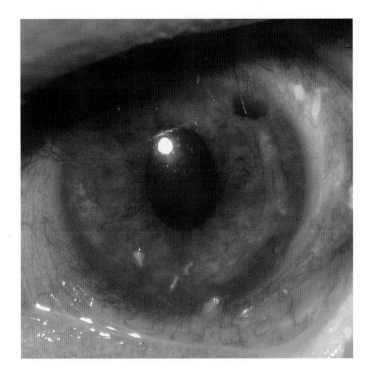

Figure 8-7 *Brownish vertical band of pigmentation on the endothelium (Krukenberg spindle) starting from the center of the pupil and extending inferiorly. Incidentally, the corneal filaments on the inferior half of the cornea are highlighted by the use of fluorescein dye.*

STEROID-INDUCED GLAUCOMA

HISTORY

- Steroid use (by any route)
- Presence of disease treated with steroids
- Usually no ocular symptoms

FINDINGS

- Elevated IOP
- Glaucomatous optic nerve in chronic cases

TREATMENT

- Discontinue use of the corticosteroid, reduce the frequency of administration, or change to a less potent steroid or steroid-sparing agent if possible
- Medical management of elevated IOP

FOLLOW UP

Contact ophthalmologist by telephone to discuss medical management and follow up.

PEARLS

Usually requires several weeks to months of steroid use before glaucoma develops. Patients using oral or topical steroid preparations more commonly develop this condition.

ICD-9 CODE

365.31   Glaucoma associated with corticosteroid use

Chapter 9

RETINA AND VITREOUS

RASHID TAHER

ANDREW WOLDORF

FLASHES AND FLOATERS

HISTORY

- Small specks or clouds moving in the field of vision; floaters can have different shapes: little dots, circles, lines, clouds, or cobwebs
- Flashes of light, often described as lightning, may appear in the periphery for several weeks or months; on rare occasions, however, light flashes may accompany a large number of new floaters and even partial loss of side vision
- The flashing lights tend to occur in only one eye at a time and persist even when the eye is closed
- History of previous retinal detachment

OTHER CAUSES OF FLOATERS

Asteroid Hyalosis

- Common degenerative process of the vitreous
- Usually found in patients older than 60 years
- Multiple, yellowish-white particles composed of calcium phosphate soaps suspended in the vitreous (Fig. 9-1)

- Asymptomatic
- Unilateral (75 percent);
- Associated with diabetes mellitus (30 percent)

Cholesterosis Bulbi

- Cholesterol crystals in vitreous
- Following a longstanding vitreous hemorrhage
- Opacities move freely inside the vitreous cavity
- Usually unilateral

Systemic Primary Amyloidosis

- Bilateral involvement with autosomal dominant familial amyloidosis
- Gradual vitreous opacification in younger patients
- Floaters are granular, glass–wool opacities
- Not associated with sudden visual loss

Vitritis

- May mimic vitreous hemorrhage obscuring the view of the retina
- Whitish cellular infiltration of the vitreous
- May be diffuse or concentrated adjacent to foci of retinitis

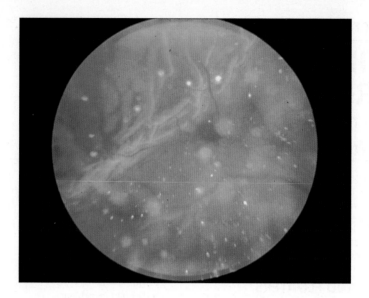

Figure 9-1 *Multiple discrete, whitish-yellow particles seen floating in the vitreous. Incidentally, a retinal detachment is also visible.*

FINDINGS ON EXAMINATION

- Decreased visual acuity accompanied by flashes and floaters are associated with vitreous hemorrhage or retinal detachment
- Feathery ring (Weiss ring) floating in the vitreous cavity if flashes and floaters associated with posterior vitreous detachment; this can be visualized with direct ophthalmoscope using the "plus" lenses

LESS COMMON

- Pigment in the vitreous (Shafer's sign)—pathognomonic for a retinal tear
- Retinal tears
- Retinal detachment

EXAMINATION OUTLINE

A complete eye examination is indicated for both eyes. Examining the uninvolved eye can provide clues to the underlying cause of flashes or floaters in the involved eye.

- Check visual acuity
- Conduct an external examination for signs of trauma
- Check confrontational visual field
- Check pupils and determine presence or absence of an afferent pupillary defect; a fixed, dilated pupil may indicate previous trauma

- Slit lamp examination: check for presence or absence of pigment in the vitreous (i.e., Shafer sign)–pathognomonic for a retinal tear in 70 percent of cases with no previous eye disease or surgery; fresh blood is identified by adjusting the slit beam tangentially and viewing the anterior vitreous directly behind the lens
- After instilling a drop of topical anesthetic, check intraocular pressure measurement in both eyes; hypotony of at least 4 to 5 mm Hg compared with the opposite eye is common in patients with a retinal detachment; however, the eye with a retinal detachment can occasionally have an increased intraocular pressure
- Conduct fundus examination with ophthalmoscopy (pupils must be dilated): direct ophthalmoscopy can detect vitreous hemorrhage and large detachment of the posterior pole, but is inadequate for complete examination because of the reduced field of view and illumination; old hemorrhage undergoes syneresis (degeneration), loses color (turns whitish yellow), and settles inferiorly; the detached retina may undulate; shallow detachments are much more difficult to detect

WORK UP

Laboratory studies are unnecessary. B-scan ultrasound may be helpful in identifying shallow or peripheral detachments.

FOLLOW UP

- Referral to an ophthalmologist for a dilated funduscopic examination should be made within 48 to 72 h of presentation
- The patient should be counseled to seek emergent ophthalmic follow up if there is a decrease in vision, increased intensity or duration of the flashes, increased quantity of the floaters, or a shadowing or loss of visual field

ICD-9 CODE

379.24   Vitreous floaters

PEARLS

- A sudden increase in floaters is a common symptom of a posterior vitreous detachment (PVD), whereby the vitreous gel pulls away from the back of the eye.

- PVD is more common in women and in myopic people, occurring 10 years earlier than in those with emmetropia and hyperopia.

- The most common complaint of patients with PVD is "floaters."

- Flashes and floaters are generally a result of vitreoretinal traction and are considered by most to signify a higher risk of retinal tears.

- Flashes of light that appear as jagged lines or "heat waves," often lasting 10 to 20 min and present in both eyes, are more likely to be a migraine. These fortification lines may or may not be followed by a headache. Visual function returns to its premigraine baseline.

- Visual loss that does not return to baseline should be evaluated for other etiologies including embolic or occlusive vascular diseases.

VITREOUS HEMORRHAGE

HISTORY

- Painless loss of vision that may be dramatic and profound
- Hundreds of tiny black specks appearing before the eye (pathognomonic for vitreous hemorrhage) resulting from disruption of a retinal vessel due to a retinal tear, mechanical traction of a vitreoretinal adhesion, or abnormal, newly formed vessels
- Moderate hemorrhage can be described as one or more dark streaks that subsequently break up into numerous, minute black spots
- Visual obstruction changes with eye or head movement
- Flashing lights can be associated with vitreous hemorrhage
- Determine use and frequency of aspirin and/or other anticoagulants
- Determine history of diabetes, sickle cell disease, retinal vaso-occlusive disease
- Determine history of head trauma and/or headaches preceding the onset of vitreous hemorrhage

FINDINGS ON EXAMINATION

- Decreased visual acuity—can be mildly impaired or decreased to light perception
- Neovascularization of the disk and/or elsewhere on the retina
- Ability to resolve retinal detail inversely correlates with the severity of vitreous hemorrhage (Fig. 9-2)

LESS COMMON

- Decreased intraocular pressure (if retinal detachment present)
- Increased intraocular pressure (if secondary to ghost cell glaucoma; see section "Treatment")
- Hyphema—in absence of trauma may indicate iris neovascularization—requires prompt ophthalmologic evaluation

EXAMINATION OUTLINE

A complete eye examination is indicated for both eyes. Examining the uninvolved eye may provide clues to the underlying cause of hemorrhage in the involved eye.

- Check visual acuity
- Conduct an external examination for signs of trauma
- Check confrontational visual field
- Check pupils and determine presence or absence of an afferent pupillary defect; a fixed, dilated pupil may indicate previous trauma
- Slit lamp examination: check for pigment in the vitreous (Shafer's sign); fresh blood is identified by adjusting the slit beam tangentially and viewing the anterior vitreous directly behind the lens
- After instilling a drop of topical anesthetic, check intraocular pressure measurement in both eyes
- Conduct dilated fundus examination with ophthalmoscopy: direct ophthalmoscopy can detect vitreous hemorrhage and large retinal detachment that involves the posterior pole but is inadequate for complete examination because of the small field of view and weaker illumination; old hemorrhage undergoes syneresis (degeneration), loses color (red blood changes to a whitish-yellow color), and settles inferiorly

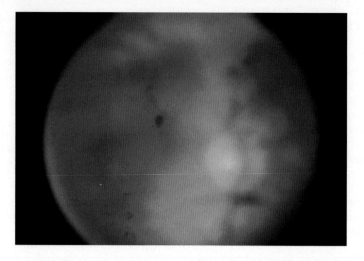

Figure 9-2 *Vitreous hemorrhage in a patient with proliferative diabetic retinopathy and neovascularization. The free-floating hemorrhage obscures the details of the retinal vessels and optic nerve.*

CHAPTER 9 RETINA AND VITREOUS

WORK UP

LABORATORY STUDIES No specific laboratory tests are necessary to diagnose vitreous hemorrhage. Testing to determine underlying medical conditions may be necessary once the etiology of the hemorrhage is determined.

IMAGING STUDIES When the view of the fundus is obstructed by hemorrhage, corneal opacification, or cataract, B-scan ultrasonography is used to confirm that the retina is attached, if an intraocular foreign body is present, and/or if a posterior vitreous detachment exists. Patients with associated neurologic symptoms (such as headache or altered mental status) may require neuroimaging to evaluate for subdural or subarachnoid hemorrhages.

TREATMENT

- Secondary or "ghost cell" glaucoma occurs if the red blood cells enter the anterior chamber and block the trabecular meshwork, resulting in elevated intraocular pressure
- If the intraocular pressure is increased, then ocular antihypertensive therapy should be considered
- If retinal and/or vitreous hemorrhage occurs in association with subarachnoid or subdural hemorrhage (Terson's syndrome), urgent neurosurgical consultation is required
- Emergent ophthalmology consultation is required if the vitreous hemorrhage has resulted from trauma or abuse, or if a retinal tear or detachment is suspected

FOLLOW UP

- For vitreous hemorrhage related to medical conditions, such as diabetes, peripheral neovascularization, or sickle cell disease, obtain a consultation within 48 h and manage the patient as an outpatient

- Discharge instructions should include limitation of physical activity and elevation of the head of the bed to 45° or more while sleeping
- Counsel patients to avoid exertional activities, heavy lifting, and aspirin-containing compounds or blood thinners
- Except in the cases of trauma and retinal detachment, close observation for 1 to 2 weeks allows time for spontaneous clearing of the hemorrhage
- Vitrectomy surgery can be helpful for patients with persistent vitreous opacities

PEARLS

- The most common cause of vitreous hemorrhage in adults is proliferative diabetic retinopathy (39 to 54 percent).

- Trauma is the leading cause of vitreous hemorrhage in people under the age of 30.

- Other major causes include retinal break without detachment (12 to 17 percent), posterior vitreous detachment (7.5 to 12 percent), rhegmatogenous retinal detachment (7 to 10 percent), and retinal neovascularization from branch or central retinal vein occlusion (3.5 to 10 percent).

- About one third of patients with intracranial (subarachnoid) hemorrhage have associated intraocular hemorrhage, and about 6 percent will have vitreous hemorrhage (referred to as Terson's syndrome).

ICD-9 CODE

379.23   Vitreous hemorrhage

RETINAL DETACHMENT (RD)

HISTORY

- A progressively enlarging dark curtain or shadow in one eye starting in the peripheral or side vision and eventually spreading to the central vision
- Initial shower of black spots, then cobwebs and dark strands in vision that result from blood in the vitreous
- Bullous (large ballooning) detachments produce dense visual field defects (blackness); flat detachments produce relative field defects (grayness)
- Waviness or distortion of a visual image (metamorphopsia) caused by fluid disrupting the normal position of the retina within the macular area
- Risk factors for retinal detachment; include: previous cataract surgery, high myopia, lattice degeneration, blunt trauma, familial history of RD, certain systemic diseases such as Stickler's syndrome and Marfan's syndrome

FINDINGS ON EXAMINATION

- Decreased visual acuity
- A fixed, dilated pupil may indicate previous trauma; a positive Marcus-Gunn pupil will occur with any disturbance of the afferent pupillomotor pathway including RD
- Vitreous pigment or tobacco dust (i.e., Shafer's sign)
- Low or high intraocular pressure measurement in both eyes
- Underlying reddish retinal pigment epithelium (RPE) and choroid more visible through tears in the retina (Fig. 9-3)
- Obvious detachment is seen as marked elevation of the retina, which appears gray with dark blood vessels that may lie in folds (Figs. 9-4 and 5)
- Comparison of the suspected area with an adjacent normal quadrant is helpful to detect any change in retinal transparency

LESS COMMON

- An orange-peel appearance (peau d'orange) of the retinal surface
- A pigmented or nonpigmented line may demarcate the limit of a detachment

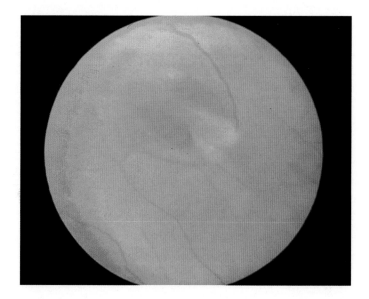

Figure 9-3 *The reddish choroid is visible through two oval-shaped tears in the retina. The brownish demarcation line superior to the break indicates that this tear has been present for a long time.*

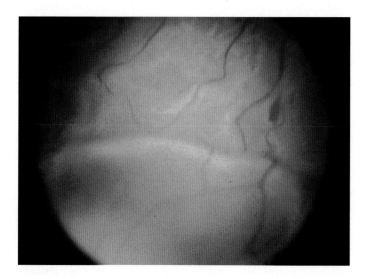

Figure 9-4 *Large, elevated retinal detachment inferiorly. Adjacent to the bullous detachment is a shallower detachment with the retina thrown into undulating folds.*

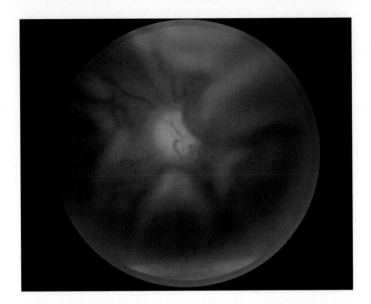

Figure 9-5 *Total retinal detachment. The detached retina is grey and thrown into multiple folds. The optic nerve can be seen centrally as the pinkish disk.*

EXAMINATION OUTLINE

A complete eye examination is indicated for both eyes. Examining the uninvolved eye may provide clues to the underlying cause of the retinal detachment in the involved eye.

- Check visual acuity
- Conduct an external examination for signs of trauma
- Check confrontational visual field
- Check for metamorphopsia with Amsler grid testing
- Check pupils and determine presence or absence of an afferent pupillary defect; a fixed, dilated pupil can indicate previous trauma
- Slit lamp examination and check for presence or absence of pigment in the vitreous (i.e., Shafer's sign)
- After instilling a drop of topical anesthetic, check intraocular pressure measurement in both eyes
- Conduct fundus examination with ophthalmoscopy (pupils must be dilated): direct ophthalmoscopy can detect vitreous hemorrhage and large detachment of the posterior pole, but is inadequate for complete examination because of the degree of magnification and poorer illumination; the detached retina may undulate; shallow detachments are more difficult to detect

WORK UP

ULTRASONOGRAPHY If the retina cannot be visualized because of corneal changes, cataracts, or hemorrhage, both A- and B-scan ultrasound can help diagnose RD and differentiate it from posterior vitreous detachment. Ultrasonography can help differentiate rhegmatogenous from nonrhegmatogenous detachment. This examination is sensitive and specific for RD but is not helpful in the localization of occult retinal breaks.

TREATMENT

When diagnosed or suspected, retinal detachment requires emergent ophthalmology consultation to confirm the diagnosis and treat the cause.

- Scleral buckle: a silicone band is sutured to the external surface of the sclera. The buckle counteracts the forces that are pulling the retina away from its normal position.
- Pneumatic retinopexy: an expanding gas bubble is injected into the vitreous cavity and the patient is positioned so that the bubble closes the retinal break allowing for the resorption of subretinal fluid. Laser or cryotherapy is used to close the tear in the retina.
- Vitrectomy: this operation removes the formed vitreous gel as well as any scar tissue or blood that has accumulated.
- Inflammatory retinal detachments usually are treated medically.

Protecting the globe in cases of traumatic retinal detachment can be important to prevent extrusion of intraocular contents (uveal tissue). Cover the eye with goggles or a metallic eye shield, if available. Avoid pressure on the globe.

FOLLOW UP

PROGNOSIS Prognosis is related inversely to the degree of macular involvement and the length of time the retina has been detached.

Surgery is the only treatment for an established retinal detachment. The goal of each operation is to relieve the retinal traction and close the retinal tears. The area around the tear is treated with cryotherapy or laser. The surgery usually consists of one or more of the following procedures.

ICD-9 CODE

361.00   Retinal detachment

- When a patient has an extensive detachment, inquiring about the initial symptoms of the visual field loss is helpful to assist in localization of the tear. Inferior field loss, which correlates with superior detachment, is the most rapidly progressive.

- The majority of retinal detachments are caused by traction from the vitreous, creating tears in the retina at the point of vitreoretinal adhesion.

- Fluid from liquid vitreous flows through a tear and separates the retina away from the underlying choroid. Because much of the blood supply to the retina is from the choroid, the retina becomes anoxic and hypofunctional when detached. If detachment is prolonged, the photoreceptor cells (rods and cods) will degenerate.

- The causes of retinal detachment can be divided into three main categories.

  1. Rhegmatogenous (*rhegma*, from the Greek word for tear) retinal detachment: due to a retinal break or tear that allows the liquid vitreous to pass through the break and·detach the retina. This is the most common type of detachment.

  2. Exudative retinal detachment: due to leakage from under the retina, which creates fluid (exudate) that detaches the retina. Many conditions can cause an exudative detachment including tumors, inflammatory disorders, connective tissue diseases, and macular degenerative conditions.

  3. Traction retinal detachments: due to pulling on the retina usually from fibrovascular tissue within the vitreous cavity. Proliferative diabetic retinopathy and proliferative vitreoretinopathy (PVR) are common causes of traction retinal detachments.

- Ten to fifteen percent of patients with symptomatic posterior vitreous detachments will have a retinal tear; if there is an associated vitreous hemorrhage, the incidence increases to 70 percent.

- Estimates reveal that 15 percent of people with retinal detachments in one eye will develop detachment in the opposite eye.

DIABETIC RETINOPATHY

HISTORY

- Refractive changes (blurry vision) with fluctuating blood glucose levels
- Mild loss of vision from macular edema and microvascular changes
- Dramatic loss of vision from neovascularization with vitreous hemorrhage and tractional retinal detachment
- History of previous laser treatment for retinopathy
- Early cataract formation associated with diabetes
- Recent cataract surgery or pregnancy associated with worsening of retinopathy
- Number of years with diabetes; increased prevalence of diabetic retinopathy associated with duration of diabetes
- Poorly controlled diabetic disease
- Associated with other diabetic complications (cardiovascular disease, stroke, diabetic nephropathy, peripheral vascular disease)

FINDINGS ON EXAMINATION

NONPROLIFERATIVE DIABETIC RETINOPATHY (NPDR) (FIG. 9-6)

- Early cortical and posterior subcapsular cataract
- Dot and blot intraretinal hemorrhages
- Retinal edema (cotton–wool spots)
- Hard exudates—yellowish deposits in the retina
- Dilation of retinal veins
- Intraretinal microvascular abnormalities (IRMA)
- Arteriolar abnormalities
- Retinal capillary nonperfusion and dropout

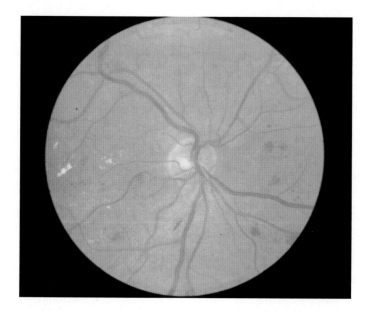

Figure 9-6 *Nonproliferative diabetic retinopathy (right eye). Multiple dot and blot retinal hemorrhages are scattered around the disk. Toward the left in the macular area are yellowish exudates due to leakage from macroaneurysms.*

PROLIFERATIVE DIABETIC RETINOPATHY (PDR) (FIG. 9-7)

- Formation of new, abnormal blood vessels
  1. Extraretinal fibrovascular proliferation (NVE)
  2. Neovascularization of the optic nerve (NVD)
  3. Neovascularization of the iris (NVI)
  4. Neovascularization of the angle (NVA)

- Vitreous hemorrhage
- Retinal traction, breaks, and detachment resulting from contraction of fibrovascular proliferation
- High intraocular pressure from neovascular glaucoma

EXAMINATION OUTLINE

- Visual acuity: cataract and macular edema can cause mild to moderate decrease in vision; vitreous hemorrhage can cause a sudden, dramatic decrease in vision
- Check reactivity of pupil with bright light
- Intraocular pressure
- Undilated slit lamp examination looking for iris neovascularization
- Undilated gonioscopy by ophthalmologist looking for neovascularization of the angle
- Dilated slit lamp examination by ophthalmologist using 60, 78, or 90 diopter indirect lenses or hand-held contact lens to assess degree of retinopathy
- Examination of peripheral retina by ophthalmologist with indirect ophthalmoscope and 20 diopter lens
- Fasting blood sugar, glucose tolerance test if no previous diagnosis of diabetes
- Check blood pressure
- Fundus photography
- Fluorescein angiogram by ophthalmologist to evaluate extent of retinal microangiopathy
- Photography to document disease

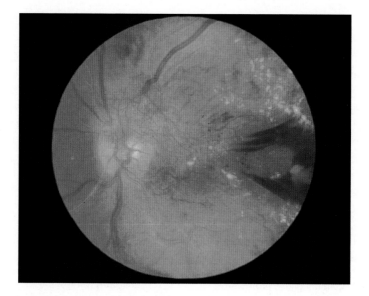

Figure 9-7 *Proliferative diabetic retinopathy (left eye). Large fronds of new blood vessels superior and temporal to optic nerve proliferate into the vitreous. The large, dark red hemorrhage overlies the background of yellowish retinal exudates and retinal hemorrhages.*

TREATMENT

Referral to ophthalmologist within several weeks for evaluation and management.

FOLLOW UP

Close follow up of diabetic patients with an ophthalmologist. All diabetic patients should be seen by an ophthalmologist at least once a year. If a patient has known diabetic retinopathy, they should be seen by an ophthalmologist more frequently.

ICD-9 CODES

250.0 Diabetes, without mention of complications
250.5 Diabetes, with ophthalmic manifestations
362.01 Diabetic retinopathy, nonproliferative
362.02 Diabetic retinopathy, proliferative

PEARLS

- Intensive insulin therapy has been shown to delay the onset and slow the progression of diabetic retinopathy, nephropathy, and neuropathy in type 1 diabetics.

- After 20 years of diabetes, 99 percent of patients with insulin-dependent diabetes mellitus (IDDM) and 60 percent with non-insulin-dependent diabetes mellitus (NIDDM) have some degree of diabetic retinopathy.

- Children less than 10 years of age are rarely found to have diabetic retinopathy.

- Pregnant patients with diabetes prior to gestation may develop diabetic retinopathy or experience progression of their diabetic retinopathy during their pregnancy. Pregnant patients with diabetes should have a baseline examination in the first trimester and repeat examination in the third trimester.

- Diabetic retinopathy is the leading cause of blindness in patients aged 20 to 64 years.

- Mucormycosis should be suspected in any diabetic who develops orbital cellulitis. An emergency computed tomography (CT) scan of the sinuses, orbit, and brain, and tissue biopsy should be performed if mucormycosis is suspected.

CENTRAL RETINAL ARTERY OCCLUSION AND BRANCH RETINAL ARTERY OCCLUSION

HISTORY

- Sudden, painless vision loss in one eye; patients report waking with no vision in one eye
- Previous episodes of vision loss lasting a few seconds to minutes (amaurosis fugax)
- History suggestive of temporal arteritis (headache, scalp tenderness, fever, arthritis, jaw claudication, weight loss, malaise)
- History of cardiac or carotid disease, use of injectable drugs (sources of embolism)
- Illicit drug history, particularly use of crack and cocaine
- Coagulopathies (polycythemia, antiphospholipid syndrome, malignancy, use of oral contraceptives)
- Trauma, such as long bone fractures, causing fat embolism
- Migraine
- Syphilis
- Sickle cell disease

FINDINGS ON EXAMINATION

- Visual acuity usually in the counting-fingers to hand-motion range
- A temporal island of vision may remain intact
- Afferent pupillary defect
- External eye appears white, without redness or tearing
- Retinal whitening with obscuration of underlying choroidal vascular pattern (Fig. 9-8)
- Cherry-red spot present in the fovea
- Segmentation of the blood column in retinal arterioles (boxcarring)
- Visualization of emboli sometimes seen at the bifurcation of retinal arterioles; emboli are typically made up of calcium, cholesterol, or platelet-fibrin (Fig. 9-9)
- Central island of good vision may remain if the macula receives blood supply from the unaffected choroidal circulation (cilioretinal artery)

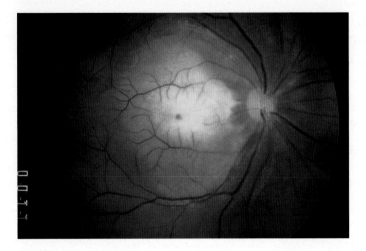

Figure 9-8 *Striking photo of a central retinal artery occlusion in a pigmented patient. The white retina obscures the underlying choroidal details. The cherry-red spot in the macula is highlighted because the whitened retinal nerve fiber layer is thinnest in this area.*

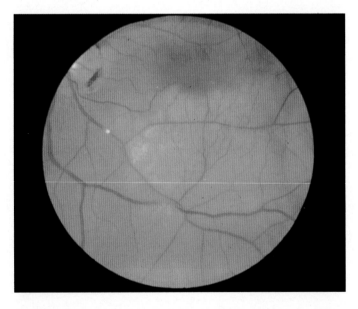

Figure 9-9 *The yellowish intra-arterial embolus (Hollenhorst plaque) interrupts perfusion of the distal wedge of retina. The anoxic retina becomes white and opacified compared with the normal adjacent retina.*

EXAMINATION OUTLINE

- Visual acuity
- Pupil testing with very bright light
- Slit lamp examination
- Intraocular pressure
- Dilated fundus examination—look for cherry-red spot, areas of retinal whitening
- Check blood pressure
- Laboratory testing: fasting blood sugar, complete blood count (CBC) with differential and platelets, lipid profile, plasma thromboplastin (PT), and partial thromboplastin time (PTT). Consider serum protein electrophoresis, hemoglobin electrophoresis, antiphospholipid antibodies, antinuclear antibodies (ANA), rheumatoid factor, fluorescent treponemal antibody absorption (FTA-Abs) test and erythrocyte sedimentation rate (ESR).
- Carotid artery evaluation: listen for bruits, duplex scan of carotid arteries
- Cardiac evaluation (echocardiogram, Holter monitor)

TREATMENT

- Immediate ophthalmic consultation
- Treatments are aimed at dislodging the embolism downstream from the occlusion site, but are generally ineffective
- Ocular massage can be started by the emergency room department while waiting for the ophthalmologist; a finger is used to alternately depress, then release the eyeball through the closed eyelid
- Intraocular pressure lowering medications can be administered by the emergency department; it is suggested that an ophthalmologist first be consulted and findings discussed before beginning these medications; acetazolamide 500 mg IV or 500 mg po and/or topical timolol 0.5% or levobunolol 0.5%

- Anterior chamber paracentesis can be performed by an ophthalmologist
- Inhalation therapy with carbogen (a combination of oxygen and carbon dioxide) can be tried since elevated Pco_2 causes vasodilation
- If giant cell arteritis is suspected, intravenous or oral corticosteroid therapy should be started immediately to prevent artery occlusion in the opposite eye
- Newer treatments by surgical or pharmacologic thrombolysis have been reported with varying successes

FOLLOW UP

- Close follow up by an ophthalmologist to look for iris, optic nerve, or retinal neovascularization; 18 percent develop ocular neovascularization, which may result in a painful glaucoma and loss of the eye
- Evaluation by an internist to complete medical work up

PEARLS

- Giant cell arteritis should be considered in all patients over 55 years of age with central retinal artery occlusion. Check for elevated ESR or C-reactive protein (CRP); perform temporal artery biopsy if suspicion is high.

- In patients under 30 years of age, the leading systemic associations are coagulopathies, migraine, and collagen vascular disease.

ICD-9 CODES

362.31   Central retinal artery occlusion
362.32   Branch retinal artery occlusion

CPT CODE

65805   Anterior chamber paracentesis

CENTRAL RETINAL VEIN OCCLUSION AND BRANCH RETINAL VEIN OCCLUSION

HISTORY

- Painless loss of vision, often occurring over hours or days
- Decrease in vision on awakening that may improve throughout the day (nocturnal arterial hypotension is thought to play a role in the disease process)
- May have recurrent amaurosis fugax or blurred vision prior to presentation
- Patient may convey history of systemic and/or intraocular (glaucoma) hypertension because both are associated with vaso-occlusive diseases
- Use of oral contraceptives and/or diuretics

EXAMINATION FINDINGS

- Decreased visual acuity
- Metamorphopsia or central visual field distortion on Amsler grid testing
- Afferent pupillary defect (if the central retinal vein occlusion is ischemic)
- Optic nerve head swelling with indistinct margins
- Dilated and tortuous retinal veins
- Extensive superficial and deep retinal hemorrhages radiating outward from the optic disk and extending into the periphery in all quadrants (Figs. 9-10 and 9-11)
- Nerve fiber layer infarcts (cotton–wool spots)
- Macular edema
- Visual field deficits

LATE FINDINGS

- Neovascularization of the iris (rubeosis irides)
- Neovascularization of the optic nerve head or retina

LESS COMMON

- Elevated intraocular pressure
- Collateral vessels of the optic nerve or retina (imply an old or resolved vein occlusion)
- Anterior chamber inflammation with cell and flare
- Vitreous hemorrhage
- Exudative retinal detachment with turbid subretinal fluid
- Hyphema

UNCOMMON FINDINGS

- Exophthalmos (e.g., thyroid eye disease or orbital tumor)
- Corneal edema secondary to rapid increase in intraocular pressure
- Macroaneurysms
- Epiretinal membrane (surface wrinkling of the retina secondary to scar formation)

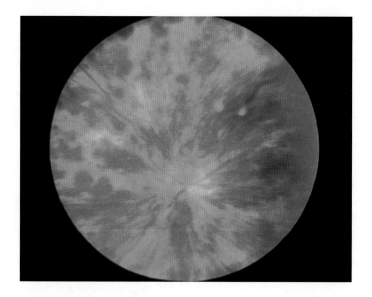

Figure 9-10 *Severe central retinal vein occlusion with retinal hemorrhages involving the whole retina.*

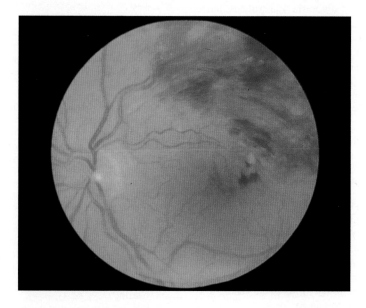

Figure 9-11 *Large retinal hemorrhages along the superotemporal vascular arcade resulting from a branch retinal vein occlusion.*

EXAMINATION OUTLINE

- Check visual acuity
- Check for metamorphopsia with Amsler grid testing; visual changes secondary to macular edema can be monitored with the grid
- Determine if there is an afferent pupillary defect
- Slit lamp examination, with special attention to determine the presence or absence of neovascularization of the iris
- After instilling a drop of topical anesthetic, check the intraocular pressure
- Check for signs and symptoms that are consistent with giant cell arteritis (including pulseless and indurated temporal arteries, jaw claudication, and scalp tenderness)
- Dilated fundus examination

WORK UP

LABORATORY STUDIES Target laboratory testing to uncover underlying medical conditions. Initial testing may include a complete blood count (CBC) and a coagulation profile to evaluate for a blood dyscrasia. Electrolytes, blood urea nitrogen (BUN), creatinine, and serum glucose also are recommended to explore the possibility of diabetes mellitus, renal disease, or dehydration. An erythrocyte sedimentation rate (ESR) can be helpful in detecting inflammatory causes and giant cell arteritis. A lipid profile can reveal an underlying hyperlipidemia. In the appropriate clinical context, a serum protein electrophoresis, or urine drug screen, could be helpful.

IMAGING STUDIES

- Chest radiograph: recommended for a complete initial evaluation; however, this may not be necessary in the emergency department.
- Fluorescein angiography: performed in ophthalmologist's office; intravenous fluorescein dye fills the retinal arterial system, but there is delayed or absent filling of the venous system (Fig. 9-12 A and B)

TREATMENT

- No effective, reliable treatment is available; however, if there is evidence of increased

intraocular pressure and/or glaucoma, then ocular antihypertensive therapy should be considered; miotics should be avoided if neovascular glaucoma is suspected or if rubeosis iridis is present
- If there is associated inflammation and/or pain (usually secondary to rubeosis iridis), topical steroids and atropine are useful

FOLLOW UP

Timely referral to an ophthalmologist.

PEARLS

- Second only to diabetic retinopathy as a cause of visual loss due to retinal vascular disease.

- Aging, high blood pressure, diabetes, smoking, and glaucoma are all risk factors.

- Less common conditions associated with vein occlusion include homocysteinemia; activated protein C resistance (factor V Leiden); protein C and S deficiency, antiphospholipid antibodies; hyperviscosity states (e.g., polycythemia and Waldenström's macroglobulinemia); inflammatory (e.g., sarcoid), and infectious (tuberculosis) conditions that cause vasculitis.

- Incidence of rubeosis among all central retinal vein occlusions (CRVOs) is about 20 percent (poor initial visual acuity is one of the strongest risk factors for development of iris or angle neovascularization).

- Neovascularization of the optic disk or retina is reported in about a quarter of ischemic CRVOs.

- About 10 percent of patients suffering from a branch vein occlusion will experience a branch or a central vein occlusion in the fellow eye in the future.

ICD-9 CODES

362.35 Central retinal vein occlusion
362.36 Branch retinal vein occlusion

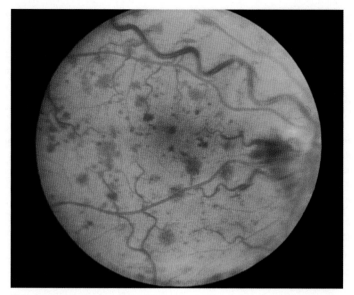

A

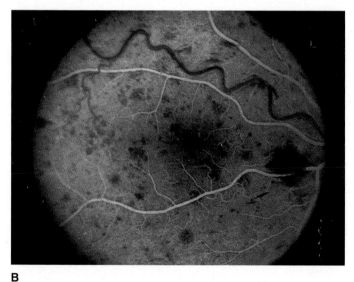

B

Figure 9-12 *A. Central retinal vein occlusion with dilated, tortuous vein superotemporal to the optic nerve. Also present are scattered dot and blot retinal hemorrhages and a flame-shaped hemorrhage at the temporal border of the optic nerve. B. Fluorescein angiography of the same patient. The retinal arterioles fill rapidly (the dye appears white on these photographs), whereas the dilated retinal veins remain dark and have blood flow.*

AGE-RELATED MACULAR DEGENERATION (ARMD)

HISTORY

- Blurred or distorted vision in one or both eyes; visual loss can be gradual (nonexudative form) or acute (exudative form)
- Distorted or wavy vision (most obvious when looking at straight lines such as doorways, telephone poles)
- Smoking history: there is an increased risk of neovascular changes
- Family history: a positive family history is a known risk factor

FINDINGS ON EXAMINATION

- Decreased visual acuity: in dry age-related macular degeneration (ARMD), mild decrease to moderate in acuity; in wet ARMD, substantial decrease usually to level of 20/400 or worse
- Metamorphopsia or central visual field distortion on Amsler grid testing
- Central or paracentral scotoma
- Light-colored irides (ARMD is uncommon in the black and Asian population)

NONEXUDATIVE (DRY) MACULAR DEGENERATION (FIG. 9-13)

- Drusen—yellowish subretinal deposits
- Macular retinal pigment epithelial mottling or atrophy

EXUDATIVE (WET) MACULAR DEGENERATION (FIG. 9-14)

- Submacular hemorrhage, yellowish exudates or serous fluid
- Submacular fibrous tissue

LESS COMMON

- Vitreous hemorrhage
- Epiretinal membrane (surface wrinkling of the retina secondary to scar formation)

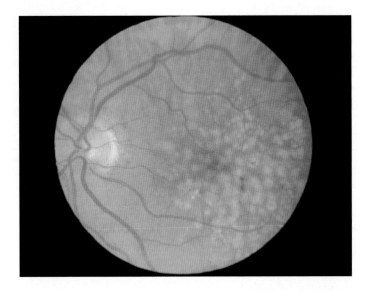

Figure 9-13 *Multiple yellowish drusen with indistinct borders are common in patients with nonexudative ARMD.*

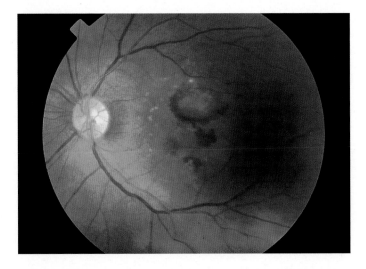

Figure 9-14 *Subretinal hemorrhage visible as the dark, grayish mass underneath the retina is a result of bleeding from new blood vessels in exudative ARMD. Visual acuity is decreased to the counting fingers level.*

EXAMINATION OUTLINE

- Check visual acuity
- Check for metamorphopsia with Amsler grid testing; visual changes secondary to macular edema can be monitored with the grid
- Determine if there is an afferent pupillary defect
- After instilling a drop of topical anesthetic, check the intraocular pressure
- Check for signs and symptoms that are consistent with giant cell arteritis (including pulseless and indurated temporal arteries, jaw claudication, and scalp tenderness) in any patient with acute visual loss
- Dilate pupils and examine fundus

FOLLOW UP

Referral to an ophthalmologist for a dilated funduscopic examination should be made within 24 to 48 h of presentation.

ICD-9 CODES

362.51   ARMD: dry
362.52   ARMD: exudative

MACULAR HOLES

HISTORY

- Loss of the central vision over a period of months
- Straight lines or objects begin looking bent or wavy (telephone poles along the roadside appear crooked, or license plates of other cars appear to have letters missing from the center of the tag)
- Reading with the affected eye becomes difficult because of the distortion of the print on the page

FINDINGS ON EXAMINATION

- Decreased visual acuity (vision is usually about 20/200 with a full thickness macular hole)
- Full confrontational fields (the peripheral vision is not affected)
- Metamorphopsia or central scotoma on Amsler grid testing
- Epiretinal membrane (surface wrinkling of the retina secondary to scar formation)
- Round retinal defect in central macula (Fig. 9-15)
- Cuff of subretinal fluid surrounding macular hole
- Yellowish deposits (drusen) in center of hole
- Round floater (operculum) in vitreous adjacent to macular hole

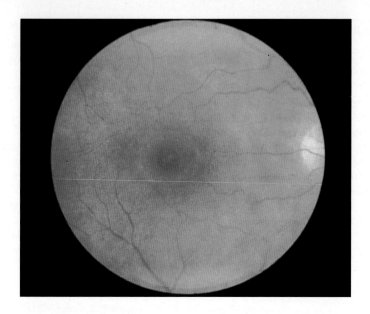

Figure 9-15 *Macular hole with cuff of subretinal fluid.*

TABLE 9-1 WATKZE–ALLEN TEST

- Orient narrow slit beam coaxial with the pupil.
- Using a 78D or 90D lens, shine thin slit at macula.
- Ask patient if there is interruption of the vertical slit beam when the slit crosses the macular hole.
- A break in the slit noticed by the patient constitutes a positive Watkze–Allen test.

EXAMINATION OUTLINE

- Check visual acuity
- Check for metamorphopsia with Amsler grid testing; visual changes secondary to macular edema can be monitored with the grid
- Determine if there is an afferent pupillary defect
- After instilling a drop of topical anesthetic, check the intraocular pressure
- Watkze–Allen test (Table 9-1)
- Dilate pupils and examine fundus

FOLLOW UP

Consultations: referral to an ophthalmologist for dilated funduscopic examination should be made within 1 week of presentation.

TREATMENT

Vitrectomy surgery has been found to successfully close between 69 and 95 percent of macular holes (the average person improves to about 20/50).

ICD-9 CODE

362.54   Macular cyst, hole, or pseudohole

PEARLS

- Macular holes are full thickness defects of the neurosensory retina involving the anatomic fovea. Although macular holes can result from trauma or inflammation of the eye, most macular holes are related to aging, occurring most commonly in the 6th to 8th decade of life.

- Macular holes are found in women twice as frequently as in men.

- Fifteen to twenty percent of individuals with a hole in one eye will later develop a macular hole in the fellow eye.

- Traction from the vitreous gel can cause the macula to be pulled apart, leaving a small round defect in the most central portion

- Individuals with a posterior vitreous detachment have a much lower risk of formation of a macular hole.

Chapter 10

ORBIT AND PLASTICS

CORINA STANCEY

SUSAN TUCKER

CONTACT DERMATITIS

HISTORY

- Any pruritus?
- How long have symptoms been present?
- Any new cosmetics or skin cleaners?
- Any new eye drops (see Table 10-1)?
- Any chemical exposure?
- Any foreign body sensation?

FINDINGS ON EXAMINATION

- Periorbital erythema; can be more prominent on lower lid and cheek
- Mild periorbital edema
- Tearing
- Thickening and lichenification of skin (Fig. 10-1)
- Conjunctival redness and inflammation

EXAMINATION OUTLINE

- Examine skin around eyes (if excessive edema, may be indicative of cellulitis)
- Check pupillary light reaction
- Check extraocular motility (if restricted or painful, may be a sign of orbital cellulitis)
- Examine conjunctiva for injection
- Look for corneal staining with fluorescein dye

TREATMENT

- Avoid contact with offending agent (may be difficult to determine exact cause)
- Cool compresses QID
- Antihistamine [naphazoline (Naphcon, Vasocon) QID] if the conjunctiva is also inflamed
- Mild steroid cream (dexamethasone 0.05 percent) to periorbital skin TID for 1 week
- Systemic antihistamine [diphenhydramine (Bendryl)] for several days if itching is severe

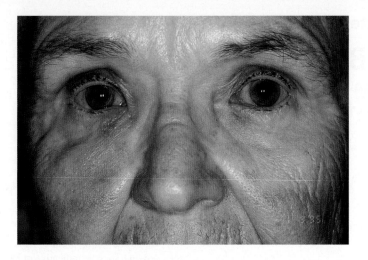

Figure 10-1 *Contact dermatitis involving the skin around the right eye. Note the unilateral redness and thickening of the periocular skin.*

CHAPTER 10 ORBIT AND PLASTICS

TABLE 10-1 COMMON OPHTHALMIC MEDICATIONS THAT CAN CAUSE CONTACT DERMATITIS

- Neomycin (sometimes found in combination with other drugs)
- Sulfacetamide
- Atropine
- Apraclonidine (Iopidine)
- Brimonidine (Alphagan)
- Preservatives (benzalkonium chloride, thiomerisol)

FOLLOW UP

- In 24 hours if suspicion of cellulitis or tissue infection
- In 1 week to ensure resolving symptoms

ICD-9 CODE

373.32 Contact dermatitis involving the eyelid

PEARLS

- Usually secondary to eye drops, cosmetics, soaps, or face lotions.

- Resolves quickly when offending agent is stopped.

- Differential diagnoses include: herpes simplex, herpes zoster, preseptal cellulitis, chemical burn, atopic disease.

PRESEPTAL CELLULITIS

HISTORY

Definition: infection involving the soft tissues of the eyelids anterior to the orbital septum and not involving the orbital structures.

- History of recent trauma? Retained foreign body?
- History of sinusitis?
- History of recent chalazion?
- History of dacrocystitis?
- How long have the symptoms been present?

FINDINGS ON EXAMINATION

- Periorbital edema and erythema (Fig. 10-2)
- Conjunctival injection
- Chemosis
- Skin tenderness, warmth
- Mild fever
- May not be able to open eye secondary to lid edema

IMPORTANT NEGATIVE FINDINGS

- No proptosis
- No ocular muscle restriction or pain with movement

EXAMINATION OUTLINE

- Check gross visual acuity
- Check for ocular motility restriction or pain with eye movement—if present, consider orbital cellulitis
- Check for proptosis—if present, consider orbital cellulitis
- Palpate lids for chalazion
- Pressure to nasolacrimal system observing for discharge
- Tap on sinuses to elicit pain secondary to sinusitis
- Vital signs (especially temperature)
- Gram's stain and culture of any open wound or drainage
- CT of the brain and orbits if there is any suspicion of orbital cellulitis

TREATMENT

- Mild preseptal cellulitis: amoxicillin–clavulanic acid (Augmentin) or cefaclor (Ceclor) for 10 d; trimethoprim–sulfamethoxazole (Bactrim) if allergic to penicillin
- For moderate to severe disease or noncompliant patient, consider IV antibiotics (Ceftriaxone and Vancomycin)
- If no improvement or worsening after several days of oral antibiotics, consider IV antibiotics
- Warm compresses QID
- Polysporin or erythromycin ointment to the eye if secondary conjunctivitis present
- Tetanus vaccine if traumatic etiology
- Exploration and debridement of flocculent mass or abscess
- Gram's stain and culture of the wound and any drainage

FOLLOW UP

- Daily until significant improvement and then every few days until resolved
- Refer to ophthalmologist for follow up

PEARLS

Infecting organisms:

- *Staphylococcus aureus* and *Streptococcus* sp. are the most common organisms.

- *Haemophilus influenzae* more common in younger children.

- Anaerobes common if foul-smelling discharge, necrosis, or history of animal/human bite.

- Viral (herpes simplex virus; herpes zoster virus) if associated with a vesicular skin rash.

ICD-9 CODE

373.13   Preseptal cellulitis

CPT CODE

67700   Drainage of abscess

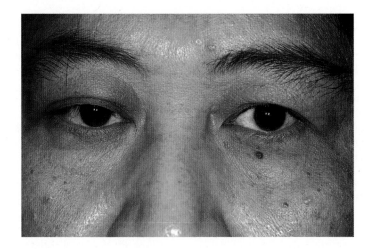

Figure 10-2 *Right eye preseptal cellulitis with mild lid edema, fullness, erythema, and conjunctival injection. The swelling causes a slight droop for the right upper eyelid.*

ORBITAL CELLULITIS

HISTORY

- Child? Immunocompromised? Alcoholic? Diabetic?
- Recent trauma? May develop months after trauma if foreign body present
- Recent chalazion? Sinusitis? Dacrocystitis? Orbital floor fracture?
- Recent dental infection?
- Recent eye surgery?
- Recent ear/nose/throat/systemic infection?
- Stiff neck or mental status changes?

FINDINGS ON EXAMINATION

- Pain and/or restriction of ocular motility
- Decreased visual acuity
- Double vision
- Periorbital edema and erythema (Fig. 10-3A)
- Conjunctival injection, chemosis
- Afferent-papillary defect
- Optic disk edema
- Proptosis (Fig. 10-3B)
- Decreased periorbital sensation
- Leukocytosis
- Fever
- Headache

If extension into cavernous sinus

- Bilateral cranial nerve II to VI palsy
- Severe edema
- Septic fever
- Nausea and vomiting
- Headache
- Decreased consciousness
- Intracranial abscess and meningitis

EXAMINATION OUTLINE

- Check visual acuity
- Check for afferent pupillary defect
- Check for ocular motility restriction or pain with movement
- Check for proptosis
- Check for decreased periorbital skin sensation
- Check vital signs, mental status, neck flexibility or rigidity
- CBC with differential, blood cultures
- Explore and debride wound if present and obtain Gram's stain and culture of drainage
- CT or MRI of orbits and sinuses (axial and coronal sections with and without contrast) to look for orbital and subperiostial abscess, foreign body, sinusitis (Fig. 10-4)
- Lumbar puncture if meningitis suspected

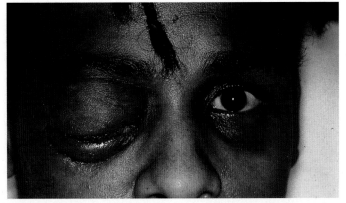

A

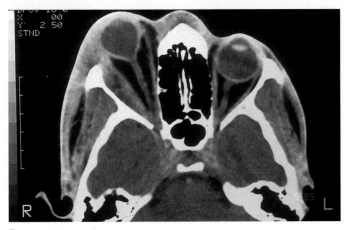

B

Figure 10-3 *A. Right orbital cellulitis caused by* Escherichia coli *and* Staphylococcus aureus. ***B.*** *CT showing right proptosis and elongation of the globe secondary to traction from swelling. Notice the temporally located subperiosteal abscess.*

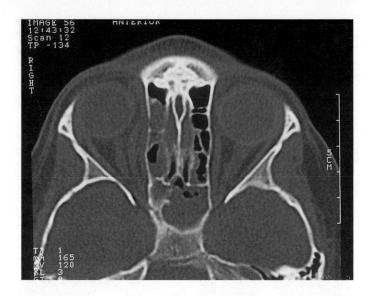

Figure 10-4 *Axial CT showing a right subperiosteal abscess displacing the medial rectus muscle.*

TREATMENT

- Admit for IV antibiotics for 1 week: ceftriaxone and vancomycin or nafcillin
- Post-traumatic or animal bites: also cover for gram-negative and gram-positive bacilli and anaerobic bacteria
- Broad-spectrum antibiotic eye drops [Trimethoprim–polymyxin B (Polytrim), ofloxacin (Ocuflox)]
- Nasal decongestants and vasoconstrictors
- Early surgical drainage of paranasal sinuses by ENT specialist if sinusitis present (more common in adults)

FOLLOW UP

- Every day while in the hospital (may take 24 to 36 h to show improvement) and every 2 to 3 d while on oral antibiotics; should be followed up by ophthalmologist
- Check visual acuity, ocular motility, temperature, and WBC daily
- Change to oral antibiotics when cellulitis is consistently improving for a 14-day total course: amoxicillin–clavulanic acid (Augmentin) or cefaclor (Ceclor)

ICD-9 CODE

376.01   Orbital cellulitis

CPT CODE

67700   Drainage of abscess

CHALAZION AND STYE

HISTORY

Definition: a subacute or chronic granuloma surrounding a blocked sebaceous or meibomian gland.

- History of previous chalazia? Previous incision and drainage?
- How long has current one been present?
- Any attempts to use hot compresses?
- Any pain present?

FINDINGS ON EXAMINATION

- Subcutaneous nodule within the eyelid (Figs. 10-5 and 10-6)
- May be palpable and visible
- Swelling of eyelid tissues around lesion
- Localized tenderness
- Erythema around lesion
- Thick, cheesy secretions expressed from meibomian gland orifice with gentle pressure
- Can also be painless
- Can extend through conjunctiva appearing as a pyogenic granuloma

EXAMINATION OUTLINE

- Palpate for eyelid nodule
- Assess area for tenderness, erythema, and edema; if extensive, may be sign of cellulitis or preseptal cellulitis
- Check extraocular motility (if restricted or painful, may be sign of orbital cellulitis)

TREATMENT

- Warm compresses QID for 15 to 20 min at a time
- May require incision and curettage if does not resolve in 3 to 4 weeks
- Intralesional steroid injection can hasten resolution of swelling and erythema

FOLLOW UP

- In 24 hours if suspicious for cellulitis
- In 1 to 2 weeks if does not resolve with warm compresses

PEARLS

- Rule out preseptal cellulitis and orbital cellulitis
- Chalazia are more common in patients with rosacea, acne, or an oily complexion
- Recurrent chalazia in the same location may actually be sebaceous cell carcinoma
- If loss of lashes present, suspect carcinoma (requires biopsy)

ICD-9 CODE

373.2   Chalazion

CPT CODES

67800   Excision of single chalazion
67801   Excision of multiple chalazia on the same lid
67805   Excision of multiple chalazia on different lids

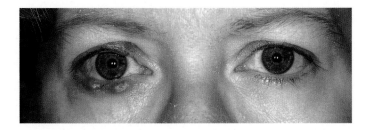

Figure 10-5 *Multiple chalazia involving the right upper and lower lids.*

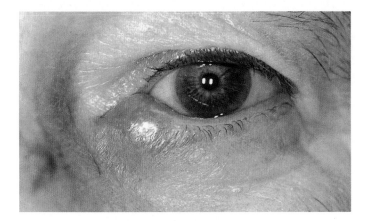

Figure 10-6 *Chalazion near the left lower lid canthal area. Lesions in this area can be mistaken for dacryocystitis.*

SKIN CANCERS

- Basal cell carcinoma
- Squamous cell carcinoma
- Sebaceous cell carcinoma
- Malignant melanoma

HISTORY

- How long has the lesion been there? (months to years are more common for malignancy)
- Has it grown rapidly or slowly?
- Age of the patient? (skin cancers are more common in the middle-aged and elderly)
- Any history of previous skin cancers (either on the eyelids or elsewhere on the body)?
- Any history of the lesion bleeding? (more common with malignancy)
- Fair skin? History of sun exposure?

FINDINGS ON EXAMINATION

- Usually asymptomatic or mildly irritating
- Skin ulceration with crusting, inflammation
- Can be nodular, indurated, flat, pigmented, scaly
- Can have loss of lashes if the lesion is near the eyelid margin
- Malignancies are usually more destructive and distort adjacent tissues

BASAL CELL CARCINOMA

- Two thirds affect the lower eyelid
- Nodular (Fig. 10-7); elevated, pink/pearly nodule with overlying telangiectatic vessels, central ulceration with rolled borders, may become pigmented and the center can bleed
- Morpheaform (Fig. 10-8); flat, indurated, yellow/pink plaque with ill-defined borders

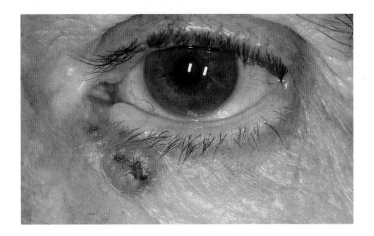

Figure 10-7 *Basal cell carcinoma of left lower lid. Pink nodule with central ulceration and rolled edges. The center appears to have bled.*

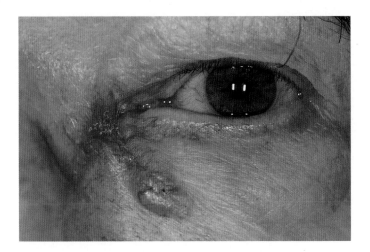

Figure 10-8 *Basal cell carcinoma of left lower lid. Morpheaform/nodular type.*

SQUAMOUS CELL CARCINOMA (FIG. 10-9)

- May appear similar to basal cell carcinoma
- Premalignant lesion (actinic keratosis) has scaly, erythematous, flat appearance
- Carcinomatous lesions are erythematous, indurated, hyperkeratotic plaques or nodules with irregular margins
- Often ulcerate and tend to affect lid margin

SEBACEOUS GLAND CARCINOMA (FIG. 10-10)

- May be misdiagnosed as a recurrent chalazion
- Firm yellow nodule
- Loss of lashes common
- Can involve both upper and lower lids (two thirds involve the upper lid)

MALIGNANT MELONOMA (FIG. 10-11)

- Either a flat macule with irregular borders and variable pigmentation, or with mild elevation and irregular borders

EXAMINATION OUTLINE

- Check skin around eye and on face for additional lesions
- Measure extent of lesion and obtain photographs prior to biopsy or excision
- Palpate preauricular and submaxillary nodes for enlargement and possible metastasis

TREATMENT

BIOPSY

- Usually incisional
- If malignant melanoma suspected, excision with wide margins

SURGICAL EXCISION

- Via Mohs micrographic surgery or frozen section control

Prior to biopsy or excision, photos need to be taken to document the exact location of the lesion in case additional tissue needs to be excised.

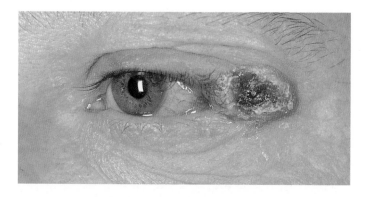

Figure 10-9 *Squamous cell carcinoma. Hyperkeratotic nodule with ulcerated center.*

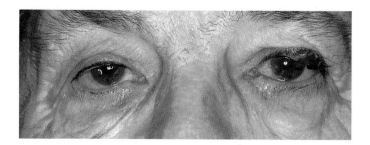

Figure 10-10 *Sebaceous gland carcinoma. Notice loss of lashes and firm nodule, which can be mistaken as a recurrent chalazion.*

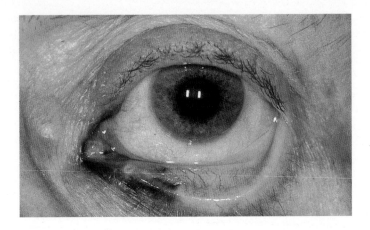

Figure 10-11 *Malignant melanoma of left lower lid. Flat lesion with irregular borders and hyperpigmentation.*

FOLLOW UP

- Every 1 to 4 weeks post-biopsy or excision until surgical site is healed
- Every 6 to 12 months looking for recurrence in same or different location

DIFFERENTIAL DIAGNOSES

- Seborrheic keratosis

- Chalazion

- Verruca—papillomatous appearance with hairs

- Keratoacanthomas appear similar to basal cell and squamous cell carcinoma but grow very quickly and then often resolve spontaneously

- Cysts are well circumscribed and have a clear or whitish fluid collection

- Molluscum contagiosum—frequently multiple with a central crater with white, cheesy material

- Nevi are light to dark brown, well circumscribed, and do not change in size

Inflammatory masses usually present with swelling, redness, and pain. Initiate medical treatment. If the lesion remains, perform biopsy or excision.

BASAL CELL CARCINOMA

- Most common malignant eyelid tumor
- Rarely metastasizes but can be highly locally invasive
- Grows very slowly

- Two thirds affect the lower eyelid
- Nodular, most common type
- Morpheaform, second most common; a more aggressive type; may be difficult to assess clinically the extent of tumor

SQUAMOUS CELL CARCINOMA

- Metastasis uncommon
- Often on sun-exposed skin
- Slow growing

SEBACEOUS GLAND CARCINOMA

- Can involve both upper and lower lids (two thirds involve the upper lid)
- Highly malignant and aggressive (can metastasize to lymph nodes and blood)
- High recurrence rate
- Excise with large borders
- Send specimen as fresh tissue for fat stains (e.g., oil red O)
- Malignant melanoma
- Can metastasize quickly to lymph nodes or liver
- Prognosis depends on the size and depth
- Excise with large borders
- If involvement of orbit, may need exenteration

ICD-9 CODES

172.1	Malignant melanoma of the eyelid
173.1	Other malignant neoplasms of the eyelid

CPT CODES

67810	Biopsy of eyelid
67840	Excision of lesion of the eyelid involving more than just skin
11640–11646	Excision of malignant eyelid lesion involving only skin

DACRYOCYSTITIS

HISTORY

- Any discharge or pain?
- Ever had similar symptoms before?
- Any recent trauma?
- Any recent nasal or sinus surgery?
- Any history of nasolacrimal duct obstruction? (excessive tearing and crusting)
- Recent ear/nose/throat infection?

FINDINGS ON EXAMINATION

- Pain and swelling over medial canthal area (Fig. 10-12)
- Erythema
- Swelling over lacrimal sac (inner/nasal aspect of lower eyelid) below medial canthal tendon
- Excessive tearing, mucopurulent discharge, crusting
- Fever
- Can develop fistula to external skin

EXAMINATION OUTLINE

- Check gross visual acuity
- Apply pressure to lacrimal sac and look for purulent discharge from the punctum; culture and Gram's stain material if present (Table 10-2)
- Check ocular motility; if restricted or painful, consider orbital cellulitis
- Check for afferent pupillary defect
- Check for proptosis of affected side
- Palpate mass for pulsation or fluctuance
- CT or MRI of orbit and paranasal sinuses for severe cases, for cases in which orbital cellulitis is suspected, or for lesions that do not respond to oral antibiotics

TREATMENT

- Oral antibiotic
  - Children: amoxicillin–clavulanic acid (Augmentin) or cefaclor (Ceclor) for 10 to 14 d; if febrile, acutely ill, or unreliable— IV cefuroxime (Zinacef, Ceftin, Kefurox)
  - Adults: cefalexin (Keflex) or amoxicillin– clavulanic acid (Augmentin) for 10 to 14 d; if febrile or acutely ill: IV cefazolin (Ancef)
- Topical antibiotic drop [trimethoprim– polymyxin B (Polytrim), ofloxacin (Ocuflox)]
- Warm compresses and gentle massage over area QID
- Incision and drainage for pointing abscesses
- In chronic cases, may need dacryocystorhinostomy with silicone intubation to bypass current drainage system

FOLLOW UP

- Daily until symptoms resolve (refer to ophthalmologist or otolaryngologist for follow up)
- If signs and symptoms worsen, admit for IV antibiotics

PEARLS

- Rule out preseptal cellulitis.

- Rule out orbital cellulitis (pain or restriction with ocular motility, proptosis, afferent pupillary defect, decreased visual acuity, intraorbital or subperiostial abscess on imaging).

- Masses above the medial canthal tendon may be mucoceles. Consider CT scanning before surgery or drainage.

- Suspect nasolacrimal gland tumor if bloody discharge from punctum.

- Can recur in 60 percent of cases.

ICD-9 CODES

375.30	Dacryocystitis, unspecified
375.32	Acute dacryocystitis
375.33	Dacryocystitis with purulent drainage
375.42	Chronic dacryocystitis
771.6	Neonatal dacryocystitis

CPT CODE

67700	Drainage of abscess

TABLE 10-2   BACTERIA CAUSING DACRYOCYSTITIS

- Acute
  Staphylococcus aureus
  Staphylococcus epidermidis
  Beta-hemolytic Streptococcus
- Chronic
  Haemophilus influenzae
  Streptococcus pneumoniae
  Actinomyces

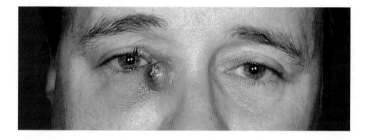

Figure 10-12   *Dacryocystitis. Large inflamed nodular area over the right nasolacrimal sac.*

PROPTOSIS

HISTORY

Definition: protrusion of the eye or eyes

- History of thyroid disease?
- History of recent trauma?
- History of cancer?
- Fever or recent infection?
- Pain with eye movements?
- Rapid or slow onset?

FINDINGS ON EXAMINATION

- Visible bulging of globe
- Lid retraction; patients have "surprised" appearance (Fig. 10-13A and B)
- Exposure keratopathy with complaints of burning, foreign body sensation, redness; irregular epithelium on inferior cornea; areas of punctate corneal erosions highlighted with fluorescein staining
- Lagophthalmos (Fig. 10-13C); incomplete eyelid closure leaving the ocular surface exposed
- Decreased vision
- Double vision
- Eyelid swelling
- Decreased extraocular motility

EXAMINATION OUTLINE

- Check visual acuity
- Check for ocular motility limitations or pain with motility
- Check visual fields and pupillary reaction to light
- Check for lagophthalmos; have patient gently close eyelids and check for any gap between upper and lower lids
- Check cornea with instillation of fluorescein dye; small punctate staining of lower one third of cornea
- Check intraocular pressure with patient looking straight ahead and in upgaze
- Check for resistance to retropulsion
- Place patient in the supine position and from above the head, look over the globes to see if they are asymmetrically displaced (one method to check for proptosis)
- Check vital signs (fever)
- Check thyroid studies and CBC
- CT or MRI of the orbits to rule out intraorbital mass if proptosis is acute

TREATMENT

For lagophthalmos or exposure keratopathy:

- Artificial tears, lubricating ointments (lacrilube), and eyelid taping at bedtime
- Surgical closure of eyelids (tarsorrhaphy) for severe exposure

If any visual field loss, optic nerve swelling, or other compressive signs, may need orbital decompression, oral steroids, or radiation for severe thyroid eye disease.

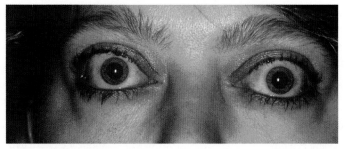

A

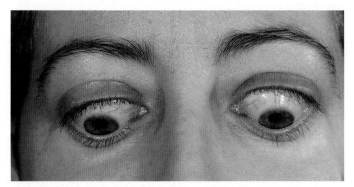

B

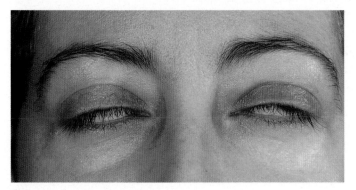

C

Figure 10-13 *A. Thyroid eye disease with exophthalmos (proptosis) and lid retraction. Note the visible sclera above and below the cornea. B. Thyroid eye disease with lid retraction on downgaze. Normally the upper eyelid margin rests at the superior limbus. C. Thyroid eye disease with lagophthalmos. The sclera is showing despite attempts to close the eyelids.*

FOLLOW UP

- Optic nerve compression (decreased vision, abnormal pupillary response) requires an urgent ophthalmology and endocrine consult
- If mild proptosis with only corneal exposure—every 3 to 6 months by an ophthalmologist

ICD-9 CODES

370.34 Exposure keratitis
374.22 Lagophthalmos
376.01 Orbital cellulitis

376.11 Orbital pseudotumor
376.21 Thyrotoxic exophthalmos
376.22 Inability to move the eye secondary to exophthalmos
376.30 Exophthalmos unspecified
376.31 Constant exophthalmos
376.35 Pulsating exophthalmos

CPT CODE

67875 Surgical tarsorrhaphy

PEARLS

ETIOLOGY

Thyroid Eye Disease

- Bilateral
- Eyelid retraction on downgaze
- Lagophthalmos
- CT shows thickening of the ocular muscle bellies without involvement of the tendons (Fig. 10-14A and B); can lead to compressive optic neuropathy if the muscles get too large

Orbital Inflammatory Pseudotumor

- Often painful
- Afebrile
- CT shows thickening of the ocular muscle bellies and tendons
- Responds dramatically to systemic steroids

Orbital Cellulitis

- Febrile
- Elevated WBC
- Pain and restriction with extraocular motility
- Sinusitis usually present on CT

Orbital and Lacrimal Gland Tumors

- Downward displacement of globe
- CT scan showing retro-orbital mass

Carotid-Cavernous Sinus Fistula

- Unilateral pulsatile proptosis
- Usually have a recent history of trauma

Cavernous Sinus Thrombosis

- Bilateral proptosis
- Fever
- Decreased consciousness

Enophthalmos of Fellow Eye after Orbital Floor Blowout Fracture (Pseudoproptosis)

- Protruding eye actually the normal position
- CT scan showing floor fracture of contralateral eye

Arteriovenous Malformation (Varices)

- Intermittent proptosis, especially with Valsalva maneuver

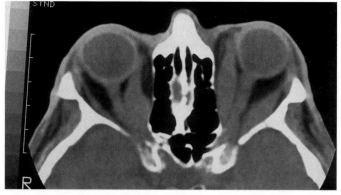

A

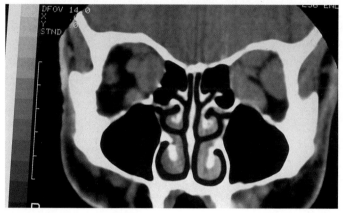

B

Figure 10-14 *A. Axial CT sections showing enlargement of the muscle bellies but not the tendons. **B.** Coronal cuts showing bilateral muscle belly thickening in thyroid eye disease leading to compressive optic neuropathy.*

CAROTID-CAVERNOUS SINUS FISTULA (C-C FISTULA)

HISTORY

- Recent trauma?
- Spontaneously occurring vs. post-traumatic (more common)
- Ocular bruit? The patient may complain of a "swooshing sound" in the ears
- Recent infection?
- Severe headache?

FINDINGS ON EXAMINATION

- Traumatic fistulas more often have high flow into the cavernous sinus from the intracavernous sinus segment of the carotid artery
- Spontaneous fistulas more commonly are low flow (Fig. 10-15); occur with atherosclerosis, hypertension, collagen vascular disease, and during or after childbirth

- Severe conjunctival congestion and dilation of conjunctival vessels (Fig. 10-16A, B, C)
- Severe conjunctival chemosis
- Pulsating proptosis (difficult to observe, but may be palpable)
- Loud bruit heard over the closed eyelid or temple with the bell of the stethoscope
- Double vision
- Eyelid droop
- Facial pain and numbness
- Restricted ocular motility on one side; CN VI most frequently affected
- Ipsilateral constricted (Horner's) or dilated pupil (if CN III involved)
- Elevated intraocular pressure
- Decreased visual acuity secondary to optic nerve ischemia or compression
- Retinal venous engorgement with dot/blot hemorrhages

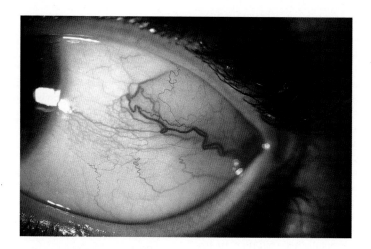

Figure 10-15 *Dilated conjunctival vessels in a patient with a direct carotid-cavernous sinus fistula.*

EXAMINATION OUTLINE

- Check visual acuity
- Check pupils for afferent pupillary defect
- Check ocular motility; may even have a frozen globe (no movement in any direction)
- Listen for bruit over the eyelid and temple with stethoscope
- Check intraocular pressure; may be elevated secondary to increased episcleral venous pressure
- Dilated fundus exam looking for dot/blot hemorrhages
- Resistance to retropulsion
- CT (axial and coronals) and/or MRI of sinuses, orbit, and brain, looking for enlarged superior ophthalmic vein (Fig. 10-16)
- Color Doppler imaging looking for reversal of flow in the ophthalmic artery
- Selective internal and external carotid artery arteriography (gold standard for diagnosis)

TREATMENT

- Fistula may close spontaneously or after arteriography
- Treat high intraocular pressure with aqueous suppressant medications (e.g., timolol)
- Selective intra-arterial embolization (requires neurosurgical/interventional neuroradiologic technique)

FOLLOW UP

Ophthalmology and neuroradiology to follow closely.

PEARLS

- Rule out cavernous sinus thrombosis (usually bilateral with fever).

- Findings are generally ipsilateral to the fistula but can be bilateral or contralateral.

ICD-9 CODES

376.35　Pulsating proptosis
747.81　Congenital carotid-cavernous sinus fistula
900.82　Traumatic carotid-cavernous fistula

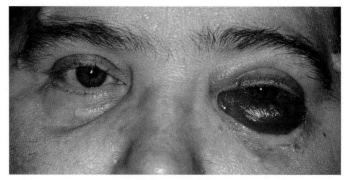

A

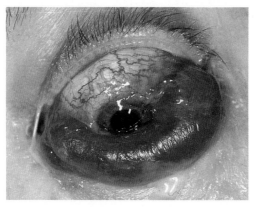

B

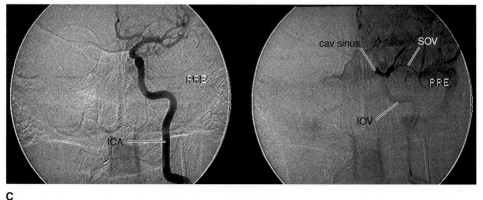

C

Figure 10-16 *A. Direct carotid-cavernous sinus fistula. Left internal carotid communication with cavernous sinus. B. Extensive conjunctival chemosis and dilated conjunctival vessels are present. Pupil is mid-dilated. C. Arteriography of carotid-cavernous sinus fistula. Left image: dye in the internal carotid artery (ICA); right image: dye in the superior and inferior ophthalmic veins (SOV and IOV) because of retrograde flow from the cavernous sinus.*

CAROTID-CAVERNOUS SINUS FISTULA (C-C FISTULA) 213

Chapter 11

NEUROOPHTHALMOLOGY

JACK A ZAMORA

VISUAL FIELD LOSS

Visual field loss can be the result of a host of different disease processes at any point along the visual pathway from the cornea to the retina, optic nerve, and occipital cortex. Because visual information travels in an organized layout, the pattern of field loss helps to indicate the location of the injury (Fig. 11-1 and Table 11-1).

TESTING

Visual field testing is achieved by showing a target in different locations in visual space. Patients indicate whether they are able to see the object (Table 11-2).

PEARLS

- Patients may report visual loss in one eye, when in fact they have lost vision in a homonymous field (e.g., the left hemifield of each eye).

- Visual field defects that respect the vertical midline can be localized at or posterior to the optic chiasm.

- Visual field defects that respect the horizontal midline are generally caused by optic nerve disease rather than retinal disease.

- The more congruous the visual field defects are, the more posterior the localization.

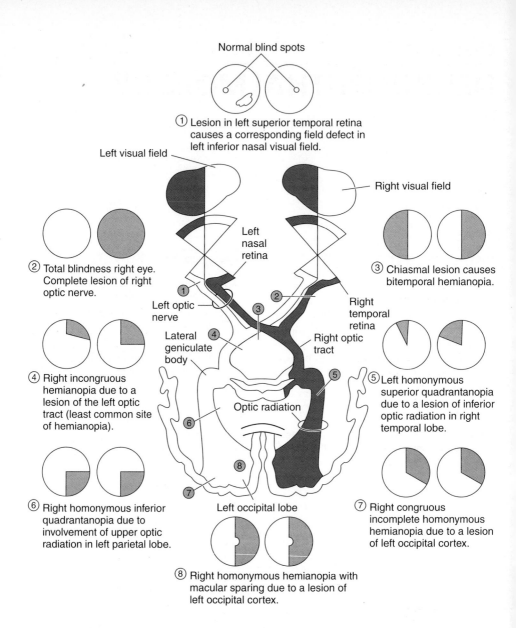

Normal blind spots

① Lesion in left superior temporal retina causes a corresponding field defect in left inferior nasal visual field.

Left visual field

Right visual field

Left nasal retina

② Total blindness right eye. Complete lesion of right optic nerve.

③ Chiasmal lesion causes bitemporal hemianopia.

Left optic nerve

Right temporal retina

Lateral geniculate body

Right optic tract

④ Right incongruous hemianopia due to a lesion of the left optic tract (least common site of hemianopia).

⑤ Left homonymous superior quadrantanopia due to a lesion of inferior optic radiation in right temporal lobe.

Optic radiation

⑥ Right homonymous inferior quadrantanopia due to involvement of upper optic radiation in left parietal lobe.

Left occipital lobe

⑦ Right congruous incomplete homonymous hemianopia due to a lesion of left occipital cortex.

⑧ Right homonymous hemianopia with macular sparing due to a lesion of left occipital cortex.

Figure 11-1 *Visual field defects due to various lesions of the optic pathways.*

TABLE 11-1   VISUAL FIELD DEFECTS AND POSSIBLE ETIOLOGY

- Binasal field defect: glaucoma (Fig. 11-2), bilateral temporal retinal disease
- Bitemporal hemianopsia: chiasmal lesion
- Blind spot enlargement: papilledema, drusen, myopia, optic nerve coloboma; b
  by formal visual field testing
- Central scotoma: macular disease, optic neuritis, advanced glaucoma
- Homonymous hemianopsia: optic tract or lateral geniculate body lesion, temporal, parietal, occipital lobe lesion (stroke or tumor) (Fig. 11-3)
- Arcuate defects: glaucoma, optic nerve disease
- Scattered focal defects: retinal pathology, media opacities
- Severe constriction of visual field with only central vision preservation: advanced glaucoma, peripheral retinal disorders, papilledema, nonphysiologic visual loss

TABLE 11-2   TYPES OF VISUAL FIELDS

- Confrontational: gross evaluation of field loss
- Tangent screen: different targets are moved in from the periphery on a black screen; the field can be measured with the patient at varying distances from the screen
- Goldmann: different-sized targets are moved centrally from the periphery to identify borders of seen/not seen areas
- Humphrey: targets are flashed in random spots in the visual field; can identify smaller, isolated defects

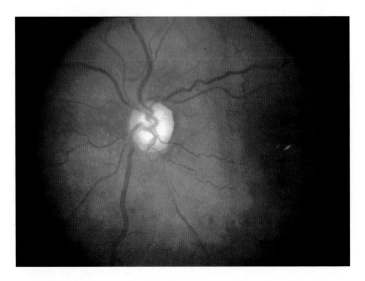

Figure 11-2 *Glaucomatous cupping and cystoid macular edema.*

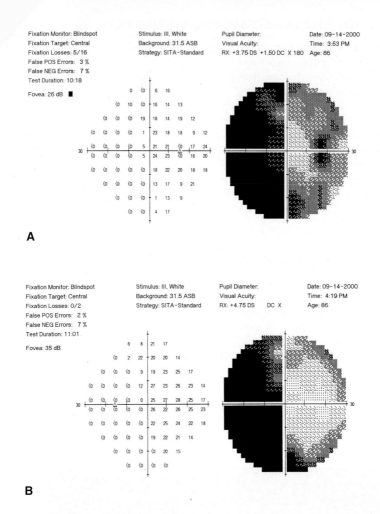

Figure 11-3 *A. and B. Humphrey visual fields for the right and left eyes of a patient with an occipital stroke. Evaluation of double vision (diplopia).*

DOUBLE VISION

Double vision (diplopia) must first be determined to be either monocular or binocular (Fig. 11-4). Test for double vision with each eye covered. If the double vision persists in one eye, then the patient is described as having monocular diplopia. If the double vision is eliminated by covering either eye, the patient has binocular diplopia.

Monocular diplopia is a result of a refractive error. This may be due to visual aberration from eyeglasses, irregularity of the cornea, or the lens. Utilizing the pinhole device on the occluder will correct monocular diplopia. Ophthalmologic examination may reveal a corneal scar, a subluxed or dislocated lens (natural or artificial intraocular lens), malpositioned surgical iridectomy, or simply crooked glasses.

ICD-9 CODE

368.2   Diplopia

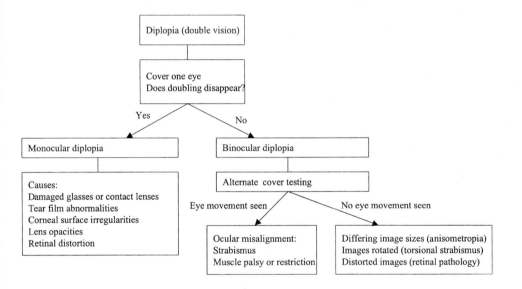

Figure 11-4 *Evaluation of double vision (diplopia).*

OPTIC NEURITIS

HISTORY

- Acute mild to severe loss of vision in one eye
- Worsening vision over course of 1 week
- Generally, young to middle-aged females
- History of multiple sclerosis, Lyme disease, or recent viral illness

FINDINGS ON EXAMINATION

COMMON

- Acute unilateral decrease in visual acuity
- Progression of visual acuity loss over 1 week
- Visual acuity does not improve with pinhole
- Decrease in color vision
- Reduction in perception of light intensity or brightness relative to unaffected eye
- Eye pain with movement
- Papilledema, may or may not be present
- Optic atrophy—evidence of previous episode of optic neuritis

UNCOMMON

- Eye redness
- Severe headache
- Mental status changes
- Other neurologic changes
- Flashes and floaters in vision
- Periorbital redness or swelling

EXAMINATION OUTLINE

- Check visual acuity at distance and near
- Recheck visual acuity with pinhole device on occluder
- Check pupils for reactivity
- Check for afferent pupillary defect (swinging flashlight test will demonstrate dilation of the pupil in the affected eye)
- Evaluate color vision, red saturation in particular
- Evaluate visual field
- Check extraocular muscle motility for pain with eye movement
- Slit lamp examination should appear normal
- Fundus examination with direct ophthalmoscope
- Vital signs—check temperature and blood pressure (malignant hypertension)
- Full neurologic examination
- Laboratory tests—CBC, Chem 7
- MRI of brain and orbits with gadolinium if first episode
- Consider lumbar puncture if intracranial process (infectious or inflammatory) is suspected

TREATMENT

- The general course is spontaneous visual recovery over weeks to months; however, intravenous steroids have been found to shorten the visual recovery period and decrease the recurrence of future episodes
- Methylprednisolone (Solumedrol) 250 mg IV QID for 72 h, then prednisone 1 mg/kg/day tapered over 11 days
- H₂-blocker ranitidine (Pepcid) 150 mg po BID
- In patients with previous diagnosis of multiple sclerosis or optic neuritis, observation; the natural history of the disease is for spontaneous recovery

FOLLOW UP

Hospitalize patient for intravenous steroids if necessary.

PEARLS

- Young children can present with a swollen optic disk with or without flame-shaped hemorrhages surrounding the optic nerve; adults present with normal disks

- Optic neuritis may be the presenting sign in patients with multiple sclerosis

- Do not give oral steroids alone as this is associated with an increase in the rate of recurrence

ICD-9 CODE

377.30   Optic neuritis

PAPILLEDEMA (see also PSEUDOTUMOR CEREBRI)

HISTORY

- Transient loss or change in the visual field lasting seconds to minutes bilaterally
- Headaches
- Nausea
- Vomiting
- Double vision
- Neurologic deficits accompanying increased intracranial pressure
- Symptoms precipitated by changes in posture

FINDINGS ON EXAMINATION

COMMON

- Bilaterally swollen optic disks—blurred disk margins (Fig. 11-5)
- Disk hyperemia
- Dilated and tortuous vessels
- Absent venous pulsations
- Retinal hemorrhages adjacent to optic nerve
- Cotton–wool spots adjacent to optic nerve
- Enlarged blind spot

LESS COMMON

- Decreased visual acuity
- Visual field defect

UNCOMMON

- Eye redness
- Flashes and floaters in vision
- Periorbital redness or swelling

EXAMINATION OUTLINE

- Check visual acuity
- Check pupils for reactivity
- Check for afferent pupillary defect (swinging flashlight test will demonstrate dilation of the pupil in the affected eye)
- Evaluate color vision
- Evaluate visual field
- Slit lamp examination—anterior segment should appear normal
- Fundus examination with direct ophthalmoscope for evaluation of disk margins
- Vital signs—check temperature (fever) and blood pressure (malignant hypertension)
- Full neurologic examination
- Laboratory tests—CBC, Chem 7, ESR
- Urgent computed tomography (CT) or magnetic resonance imaging (MRI) to rule out an intracranial process (mass effect, hydrocephalus) if other neurologic symptoms present
- Consider lumbar puncture to obtain opening pressure and to evaluate for intracranial process (infectious or inflammatory)

TREATMENT

- Any process that can increase intracranial pressure can cause papilledema (intracranial tumors, hydrocephalus from stenosis, or infectious etiology)
- Treatment is directed at the underlying cause

PEARLS

- Lack of spontaneous pulsations does not indicate high intracranial pressure as spontaneous pulsations are not seen in 20 percent of population.

- Spontaneous venous pulsations indicate an intracranial pressure of less than 180 mm H_2O.

- Papilledema occurs after 24 to 48 h of increased intracranial pressure.

ICD-9 CODE

377.00   Papilledema

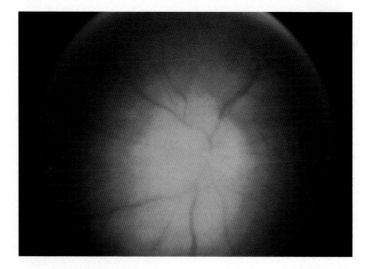

Figure 11-5 *Papilledema in the left eye of a patient. Complete obscuration of the optic nerve margin and disk vessels by the swelling of the nerve fiber layer.*

PSEUDOTUMOR CEREBRI (see also PAPILLEDEMA)

HISTORY

- Headache worse in the morning
- Transient visual field loss
- Tinnitus
- Dizziness
- Nausea and vomiting
- Stereotypically affects young, obese women

FINDINGS ON EXAMINATION

COMMON

- Overweight patient
- Optic nerve swelling (Fig. 11-6A and B)
- Visual field loss
- Decreased visual acuity
- Binocular diplopia—resolved with occlusion of one eye
- Various visual field defects possible

EXAMINATION OUTLINE

- Check visual acuity
- Check pupils for reactivity
- Check for afferent pupillary defect
- Evaluate color vision
- Evaluate visual field
- Slit lamp examination should appear normal
- Fundus examination with direct ophthalmoscope
- Vital signs
- Full neurologic examination

- MRI of orbit and brain
- Lumbar puncture
- Neurology consult

TREATMENT

- Weight loss
- Acetazolamide (Diamox) 250 mg po QID and increase as tolerated up to 500 mg QID

FOLLOW UP

See ophthalmologist within 24 h for complete evaluation.

PEARLS

- Medical history important given association with various medications (tetracycline, nalidixic acid).

- May be caused by systemic steroid withdrawal, use of high doses of vitamin A.

- Pseudotumor cerebri is a diagnosis of exclusion so laboratory studies and neuroimaging are normal.

ICD-9 CODES

348.2   Benign intracranial hypertension
377.01   Papilledema associated with increased intracranial pressure

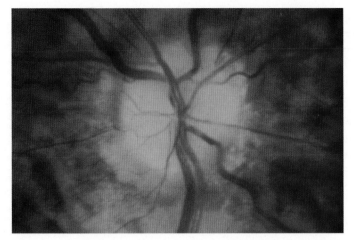

A

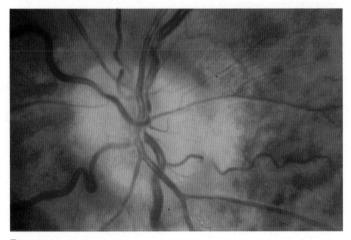

B

Figure 11-6 *High-magnification photos of the optic nerves of the right (**A**) and left (**B**) eyes in a patient with pseudotumor cerebri. Elevation and obstruction of the disk margin is more prominent in the left eye.*

ANTERIOR ISCHEMIC OPTIC NEUROPATHY

TYPES

- Arteritic—associated with temporal arteritis
- Nonarteritic—idiopathic

HISTORY

- Age greater than 51
- Acute loss of inferior or superior visual field
- Minimal to severe visual loss
- Vascular disorders: diabetes, hypertension, high cholesterol, smoking

FINDINGS ON EXAMINATION

- Normal or decreased visual acuity
- Afferent pupillary defect
- Disk swelling can be sectoral or diffuse
- Extraocular motility disorder (especially lateral movement deficit)

SIGNS OF TEMPORAL ARTERITIS

- Temporal headache
- Temporal artery tenderness
- Jaw claudication
- Scalp hypersensitivity

EXAMINATION OUTLINE

- Check visual acuity—severe loss of vision in arteritic ischemic optic neuropathy
- Check pupils for reactivity
- Check for afferent pupillary defect (swinging flashlight test will demonstrate dilation of the pupil in the affected eye)
- Evaluate color vision
- Evaluate visual field
- Slit lamp examination should appear normal
- Fundus examination with direct ophthalmoscope
- Vital signs
- Full neurologic examination
- Laboratory tests: emergent ESR, C-reactive protein, CBC, Chem 7; ESR is positive, if ESR more than (age/2) in men, or if ESR more than (age + 10)/2 in women
- Medical consult

TREATMENT

If the patient is older than 50 years of age and has an elevated ESR, treat with systemic steroids for presumptive arteritic ischemic optic neuropathy.

- Methylprednisolone (Solumedrol), 250 mg IV QID for 72 h, then slow taper *or*
- Prednisone 60 to 100 mg po qd over months to prevent ischemic neuropathy in opposite eye
- H_2-blocker ranitidine (Pepcid) 150 mg po BID

If nonarteritic, treat underlying medical condition (usually diabetes and/or hypertension). Definitive diagnosis for giant cell arteritis is with temporal artery biopsy

FOLLOW UP

If diagnosis of temporal arteritis is confirmed by biopsy, then patient is maintained on oral steroids for a period of 3 months to 1 year to suppress the disease based on symptomatology and ESR levels.

PEARLS

- If systemic steroids are not given for arteritic ischemic optic neuropathy, the contralateral eye may become affected within 24 hours.

- Associated with polymyalgia rheumatica.

- Temporal artery biopsy can be falsely negative because of patchy involvement of the artery.

- Begin steroid therapy immediately; temporal artery biopsy should be done within the first week of steroid treatment.

ICD-9 CODES

337.30   Ischemic optic neuropathy
446.5   Temporal arteritis

CRANIAL NERVE PALSY

Third Nerve Palsy

HISTORY

- Age of patient
- Hypertension or diabetes
- Time of onset
- Associated pain or discomfort
- Previous trauma

FINDINGS ON EXAMINATION

COMMON

- Inability to elevate, depress, and/or adduct eye involved
- Double vision eliminated by monocular occlusion
- Pupil may or may not be involved

UNCOMMON

- Decreased vision

EXAMINATION OUTLINE

- Check visual acuity
- Check pupils for reactivity and afferent pupillary defect
- Check ocular motility
- Slit lamp examination should appear normal
- Fundus examination with direct ophthalmoscope
- Vital signs

- Full neurologic examination, including other cranial nerves
- Emergent imaging if: (1) pupil involved: fixed, dilated, or minimally reactive, (2) patient younger than 50 years, (3) partial third nerve palsies present, (4) other cranial nerve deficits or other neurologic signs, or (5) bilateral disease.

TREATMENT

- Referral to neurology or neurosurgery
- Treatment of underlying etiology
- Patch over paretic eye for symptomatic diplopia (unless patient under 10 years of age)

FOLLOW UP

- In patients with suspected microvascular disease, follow up in 3 months
- Neurologic evaluation

PEARLS

Diabetic third nerve palsies are typically painless and spare the pupil. Ocular motility gradually returns spontaneously over 6 to 8 weeks. Imaging is indicated if the presentation is atypical or persists more than 2 months.

ICD-9 CODES

378.51   Third nerve palsy, partial
378.52   Third nerve palsy, total

Fourth Nerve Palsy

HISTORY

- Age of patient
- Duration of symptoms
- Double vision in vertical or diagonal orientation
- Recent trauma
- Hypertension or diabetes
- Difficulty reading
- May be asymptomatic

FINDINGS ON EXAMINATION

COMMON

- Weakness of depression on adduction
- Involved eye is elevated on primary gaze
- Head tilt toward contralateral shoulder to eliminate diplopia

UNCOMMON

- Decreased vision
- Light sensitivity

EXAMINATION OUTLINE

- Check visual acuity
- Check pupils for reactivity and afferent pupillary defect—pupils should not be affected in isolated CN IV palsy
- Check ocular motility
- Slit lamp examination should appear normal
- Fundus examination with direct ophthalmoscope

- Vital signs
- Full neurologic examination, including other cranial nerves
- MRI of brain when: other cranial nerve deficits or neurologic abnormalities, no history of head trauma

TREATMENT

- Emergent neurosurgical and vascular intervention if necessary
- Treatment of underlying etiology
- Patch over paretic eye for symptomatic diplopia (unless patient under 10 years of age)

FOLLOW UP

- In patients with suspected microvascular disease, follow up in 3 months
- Neurologic evaluation

PEARLS

In longstanding or congenital CN IV palsy, patients develop a head tilt away from the weak muscle and can have facial asymmetry. Review old photographs to help distinguish recent versus remote onset.

ICD-9 CODE

378.53   Fourth nerve palsy

Sixth Nerve Palsy

HISTORY

- Age of patient
- Time of onset
- Hypertension or diabetes
- Horizontal double vision
- Pain
- Recent viral infections in younger patients
- Chronic ear infections
- Recent trauma

FINDINGS ON EXAMINATION

COMMON

- Inability to move eye involved laterally
- Esotropia
- Double vision eliminated by monocular occlusion

UNCOMMON

- Decreased vision

EXAMINATION OUTLINE

- Check visual acuity
- Check pupils for reactivity and afferent pupillary defect—pupil should not be affected in isolated CN VI palsy
- Check ocular motility
- Slit lamp examination should appear normal
- Fundus examination with direct ophthalmoscope
- Otoscopic examination in children for otitis media
- Vital signs
- Full neurologic examination, including other cranial nerves

- MRI of brain when: patient younger than 50 years of age, other cranial nerve deficits or other neurologic abnormalities present

TREATMENT

- Emergent neurosurgical/vascular intervention if necessary
- Treatment of underlying etiology
- Patch over paretic eye for symptomatic diplopia (unless patient younger than 10 years of age)

FOLLOW UP

- In patients with suspected microvascular disease, follow up in 3 months
- Pediatric ophthalmology consultation to rule out amblyopia or prevent amblyopia in children less than 10 years of age

PEARLS

Most commonly secondary to trauma or microvascular disease in adult (diabetes, hypertension, atherosclerosis). In children, sixth nerve palsy is usually a result of a post-viral condition, however, increased intracranial pressure, a pontine glioma, and Gradenigo's syndrome (petrositis causing sixth and often seventh nerve palsy in children with otitis media) must be ruled out with imaging studies. Viral CN VI palsies resolve spontaneously with time.

ICD-9 CODE

378.54   Sixth nerve palsy

MYASTHENIA GRAVIS

HISTORY

- Weakness worsening during the evening or with repeated muscle usage, improved with rest
- Weakness of jaw, neck, trunk, limbs, dysphagia, dysarthria, dyspnea
- Ptosis
- Variable pattern of diplopia

EXAMINATION OUTLINE

- Check visual acuity
- Check pupils for reactivity and afferent pupillary defect
- Check ocular motility
- Measure amount of ptosis
- Slit lamp examination should appear normal
- Fundus examination with direct ophthalmoscope
- Vital signs
- Full neurologic examination, including other cranial nerves
- Laboratory tests: Complete blood count (CBC), Chem 7, anti-acetylcholine receptor antibody test, thyroid function tests, antinuclear antibody (ANA)
- Consider lumbar puncture if intracranial process (infectious or inflammatory) is suspected
- Tensilon test (Table 11-3)
- Sleep test: muscle function improved after 30 min of rest
- Ice test: muscle function improved after 2 min of ice
- Check swallow and proximal limb function to rule out systemic involvement
- CT scan to rule out thymoma

TREATMENT

- No treatment if mild symptoms
- Pyridostigmine (Mestanon) 60 mg po QID for moderate symptoms
- If systemic disease with respiratory involvement, urgent hospitalization for possible ventilatory support, IV steroids, and plasmaphoresis

FOLLOW UP

- For mild symptoms that have been present for more than a few weeks, follow up in 1 month
- For moderate symptoms requiring medication, follow up in few days to evaluate for improvement
- Systemic involvement may require hospitalization

PEARLS

Myasthenia gravis is associated with other autoimmune diseases and with thymomas.

ICD-9 CODE

358.0   Myasthenia gravis

TABLE 11-3 TENSILON TEST

Edrophonium (Tensilon) is a short-acting cholinesterase inhibitor. It permits acetylcholine to bind longer to the receptor permitting stronger muscle contraction.

1. Administer Tensilon 2 mg IV.
2. If symptoms do not disappear or decrease after 1 min, then can administer two additional 4-mg boluses.
3. A positive test is indicated by resolution of the ptosis or disappearance of diplopia.

ABNORMAL PUPILS AND ANISOCORIA

HISTORY

- Onset and duration
- History of trauma
- History of intraocular surgery
- Recent ocular examination
- Hypertension or diabetes
- Birth trauma
- Disruption on the sympathetic pathway: dislocated shoulder, apical lung tumors (Pancoast tumors), neck surgery

FINDINGS ON EXAMINATION

COMMON

- Difference in size of pupil noticed by others
- Unilateral ptosis, myosis, anhydrosis in Horner's syndrome

- Minimal or no co[...] accommodation in [...]
- Recent eye exam [...] mydriasis
- Pupil border irreg[...] matic pupil damag[...]

LESS COMMON

- Iris color changes [...]

EXAMINATION OUTLINE

- Complete ocular examination to rule out third nerve palsy or iris sphincter damage
- Evaluation of pupils under dim and bright lighting conditions
- Determine whether difference in pupils is greater in light or dark (Fig. 11-7)
- Perform cocaine or pilocarpine testing
- CBC, Chem 7, RPR
- CXR or chest CT if Horner's syndrome suspected without history of trauma
- Head CT scan if partial third nerve palsy suspected

TREATMENT
- Treat und[...]
- Refer [...] me[...]

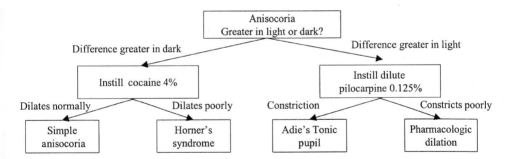

Figure 11-7 *Evaluation of anisocoria.*

...erlying cause

...o ophthalmologist for temporary treat-
...t of Adie's tonic pupil

FOLLOW UP

- Closer follow up recommended if third nerve palsy is suspected
- Otherwise, no significant follow up for anisocoria

ICD-9 CODES

337.9   Horner's syndrome
379.41   Anisocoria
379.46   Adie's tonic pupil

AFFERENT PUPILLARY DEFECT

HISTORY

- Glaucoma
- Head trauma
- Eye trauma
- Decreased vision in affected eye
- Change in color vision

FINDINGS ON EXAMINATION

- Pupils constrict with direct light
- Affected pupil may not constrict or constrict poorly
- Affected pupil dilates on swinging flashlight test (when the light moves from the normal to abnormal eye, the pupils dilate)

EXAMINATION OUTLINE

- Check visual acuity and color vision.
- Check pupils for reactivity and afferent pupillary defect in dark room with high intensity light source.
- Check ocular motility
- Slit lamp examination
- Fundus examination with direct ophthalmoscope
- Vital signs
- Full neurologic examination, including other cranial nerves
- Visual field testing

TREATMENT

- Treat underlying disease.
- Afferent pupillary defect is a sign of optic nerve damage

FOLLOW UP

- Patients with history of recent trauma may require steroids
- Outpatient follow up if patient has history of glaucoma

ICD-9 CODE

379.40   Abnormal pupillary function

MIGRAINE HEADACHE

HISTORY

- Unilateral headache, described as throbbing, aching, or pulsing behind the eyes or across the forehead (Table 11-4)
- Aura: sensations that precede migraine lasting 10 min to 1 h preceding migraine
- Visual disturbances: flashing lights, zigzag lines, blurred vision, visual field defects
- Nausea
- Vomiting
- Mood changes
- Light sensitivity

FINDINGS ON EXAMINATION

COMMON

- No specific ophthalmic findings

LESS COMMON

- Permanent neurologic deficits
- Mental status changes
- Decreased visual acuity
- Meningitic signs
- Fever
- Proptosis
- Retinal hemorrhages

UNCOMMON

- Temporary neurologic deficits

EXAMINATION OUTLINE

- Check visual acuity
- Check pupils for reactivity
- Check for afferent pupillary defect (swinging flashlight test will demonstrate dilation of the pupil in the affected eye)
- Evaluate visual field
- Slit lamp examination should appear normal
- Fundus examination with direct ophthalmoscope
- Vital signs: check temperature (fever) and blood pressure (malignant hypertension)
- Full neurologic examination
- Laboratory tests: CBC, Chem 7
- Computed tomography (CT) or magnetic resonance imaging (MRI) for complicated migraine
- Consider lumbar puncture if intracranial process (infectious or inflammatory) is suspected

TABLE 11-4   CLASSIFICATION OF MIGRAINE HEADACHES

Common	Headache without aura
Classic	Headache with aura
Acephalic or ocular	Visual aura without headache
Complicated migraine	Neurologic deficits lasting beyond headache

TREATMENT

- Bed rest in dark, low-noise environment
- Nonsteroidal anti-inflammatory agent: Ibuprofen (Motrin) 600 mg po TID; acetominophen/aspirin/caffeine (Excedrin)
- If initial therapy fails or there are greater than 3 attacks per month: ergotamine 2.0 mg po, repeat q 30 min for maximum of 6 doses per day, *or* sumatriptan (Imitrex) 25 mg po, repeat q 2 h for maximum 4 doses per day
- Prophylaxis: systemic beta-blocker (propanolol 20 to 40 mg po BID to TID); amitriptyline 25 to 75 mg po qd to BID; calcium channel blocker (Verapamil 80 mg po TID)
- Patient should be followed up by internist or neurologist

FOLLOW UP

- Refer urgently if neurologic deficits persist despite resolution of headache

PEARLS

Migraines can be triggered by many different factors: stress, caffeine ingestion, or menstrual cycles.

ICD-9 CODES

346.0	Classic
346.0	Migraine with aura
346.1	Atypical
346.1	Common
346.9	Migraine headache

Chapter 12

PEDIATRIC OPHTHALMOLOGY

MELANIE ANNE KAZLAS

KAILENN TSAO

SPECIAL CONSIDERATIONS

Examination of the eyes should begin the moment the child or infant is brought into the room. Stranger anxiety or fear of doctors may require that you complete the examination "out of order." The following are the different sections of the basic examination.

VISION

Visual acuity improves as the visual system matures and develops (Fig. 12-1; Table 12-1).

INTRAOCULAR PRESSURE

- Difficult to assess accurately in the pediatric population

- Gentle finger pressure over the eyelids, comparing one eye with the other, gives a gross indication of ocular tension
- Tono-Pen determination may be facilitated by having the mother nurse the baby during measurement
- Referral for examination under anesthesia is necessary if glaucoma is suspected

VISUAL FIELDS

Gross visual fields to count fingers are feasible in the verbal child, with patience (Fig. 12-2).

PUPIL EXAMINATION

From newborn to 1 month, the pupils of an infant are normally miotic, but pupillary reactivity and afferent pupillary defect can be checked from birth.

MOTILITY

Attempt to check fixation and following of objects in the nine diagnostic fields of gaze. If motility is not full, check movements with each eye covered. The oculocephalic maneuver may elicit horizontal gazes by rotating the child while the child maintains fixation on a point in the room.

MUSCLE BALANCE

Large deviations (Table 12-2) should be grossly quantified in each field of gaze by the Hirschberg test to check for comitance. A small ocular deviation can be confirmed with the cover test, whereupon the deviated eye will move to take up fixation as the other eye is covered.

FUNDUS EXAMINATION

Fundus examination in the poorly cooperative child is often limited to confirmation of equal red reflexes. Glimpses of the disk and macula may also be obtained with persistence at the examination. Pupil dilation is best under the supervision of the ophthalmologist. For uncooperative children examination under anesthesia is often necessary to obtain a complete eye examination.

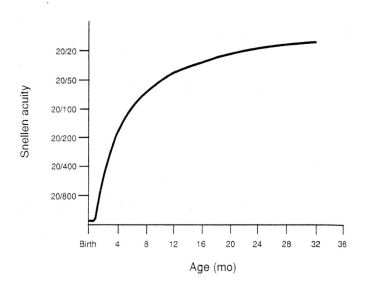

Figure 12-1 *Graph demonstrating the increase in acuity over time in the normal, full-term infant.*

TABLE 12-1 VISUAL ACUITY

Age	Expected Vision
Newborn	Blink reflex to bright light
2 mo	Fixate on a target and follow its movement
3 yr	Identify Allen picture cards or tumbling E's (Fig. 12-2)
5 yr	Snellen letter chart

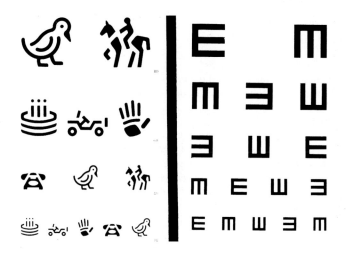

Figure 12-2 *Verbal children who do not know the alphabet may identify Allen pictures (left), or identify the direction which individual letter E points on the tumbling E chart.*

TABLE 12-2   TESTS FOR ESTIMATING DEGREE OF OCULAR DEVIATION

Bruckner test
- Have patient look at the light of the direct ophthalmoscope
- Looking through a direct ophthalmoscope at both eyes simultaneously, assess the brightness and clarity of the red reflex
- The deviated eye will have the brighter red reflex
- Useful for detecting small deviations, but does not provide quantification of degree of deviation

Hirschberg test (Corneal Light Reflex test)
- The decentration of the corneal light reflex of a penlight indicates the amount of deviation
- Deviation of 15 prism diopters (PD) for every millimeter the light reflex is displaced from the center of the pupil
- Light reflex at pupillary border = 30 PD deviation
- Light reflex at mid-iris = 60 PD deviation

Krimsky test
- Prisms are placed in front of one eye until light reflexes for both eyes are aligned
- The degree of deviation is estimated with the corrective prism

Alternate cover testing
- For cooperative patients who can fixate on a target
- An occluder is switched from covering the right eye to the left eye
- If movement of the uncovered eye is observed, place prisms in front of one eye
- Increase the strength of the prism until no movement occurs

STRABISMUS

Strabismus is manifest misalignment of the eyes with numerous etiologies and implications.

HISTORY

Much of the history can be gathered from the parents' observations

- Double vision (monocular/binocular/horizontal/vertical)—can be difficult to elicit in preverbal children
- Age of onset (congenital vs. acquired)
- Intermittent vs. constant
- Eyes turn in or out or both, or are vertically misaligned
- Patching therapy or use atropine drops
- Family history of strabismus
- Maternal history, such as maternal infection and birth history (full term or premature/traumatic/forceps/vacuum extraction)
- Past medical history (headaches, viral illnesses)
- Previous eye surgery

FINDINGS ON EXAMINATION

- Poor vision if amblyopia or a sensory cause for the strabismus
- Misalignment of eyes (Figs. 12-3 and 12-4)
- Head tilt
- Hemifacial hypoplasia toward side of tilt (congenital fourth nerve palsy)
- Nystagmus (poor prognosis)
- Abnormal pupils (third nerve palsy)
- External examination (facial deformity, trauma, telecanthus, epicanthus, limbal dermoid, masses, infection, ptosis, discoloration)
- Other physical signs (Poland anomaly, neck deformity)
- Media opacity (cataract, intraocular tumor)
- Other neurologic signs

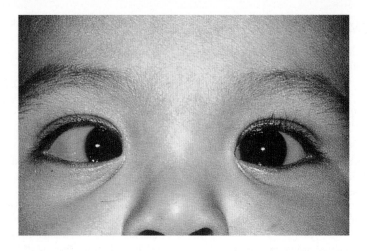

Figure 12-3 *Illustration of right esotropia, a nasal deviation of one of the eyes. The light relfex of the right eye is displaced temporally over the iris.*

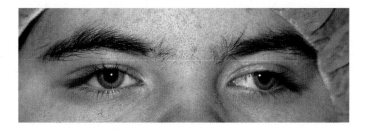

Figure 12-4 *Illustration of left exotropia, a temporal deviation of one of the eyes.*

EXAMINATION OUTLINE

- External: does the child have a constant or intermittent misalignment? does the child prefer to use one eye?
- Vision — assess each eye separately
- Pupils (red reflex)
- Motility
- Comitance and incomitance
- Hirschberg test or alternate cover test
- Intraocular pressure (IOP)
- Anterior segment
- Fundus

TREATMENT

- Expeditious referral if intraocular tumor, cataract, or sensory strabismus present
- Avoid eye patching in children under 10 years old without advice of ophthalmologist
- Treat other systemic entities as appropriate (trauma/infection, increased intracranial pressure/tumor)

FOLLOW UP

Immediacy of follow up varies according to the etiology of the strabismus.

ICD-9 CODES

378.0	Esotropia
378.1	Exotropia
378.2	Intermittent heterotropia
378.5	Paralytic strabismus
378.6	Mechanical strabismus

PEARLS

- Comitant horizontal intermittent or constant deviations, most often benign, can be referred to the pediatric ophthalmologist within a matter of days to weeks for treatment and possible amblyopia therapy. Exceptions to this are suspected cases of hydrocephalus or if there is history of double vision, whereupon neuroimaging may be prudent. Double vision is often suppressed in children under 9 years of age and will often lead to amblyopia over time. Intermittent deviations may improve or become constant over time.

- Children more than 1 month old with comitant vertical deviations should be imaged to rule out brainstem, midbrain, and cerebral pathology.

- Incomitant horizontal or vertical strabismus of new onset in children should have MR imaging to rule out intracranial processes, particularly in pupil-involving third nerve palsy. Exceptions to this may include restrictive processes such as congenital fibrosis syndrome, Brown's syndrome, or Duane's syndrome.

- Sensory strabismus. A unilateral decrease in vision can lead to a manifest ocular misalignment and should be referred more urgently to rule out media opacity or intraocular malignancy.

- Strabismus with pain, history of orbital trauma, or an obvious orbital mass may indicate an orbital process such as cellulitis, muscle entrapment, or malignancy, and should be imaged with 1- or 2-mm coronal CT cuts of the orbits and sinuses.

LEUKOCORIA (WHITE PUPIL)

HISTORY

Leukocoria is usually noticed by the parents and brought to the attention of the physician.

- Family history of eye problems (congenital cataracts, tumors)
- Maternal history (diabetes and drug use)
- Birth history (prematurity, birth trauma)
- Age of onset
- Past medical history
- Drug history
- Hearing deficits
- Pets and sandbox (exposure to toxoplasmosis or toxocariasis)
- Pain and infection

FINDINGS ON EXAMINATION

- Poor vision in affected eye(s)
- Horizontal nystagmus (poor prognosis)
- Cataract (Fig. 12-5)
- Glaucoma
- Vitreous hemorrhage
- Retinal abnormality
- Intraocular inflammation
- Intraocular mass (Fig. 12-6)
- Physical signs (stigmata of trisomy, incontinenti pigmenti)

EXAMINATION OUTLINE

- External (injection/mass/proptosis)
- Vision—decreased in affected eye(s)
- Pupils (red reflex present)
- Motility
- IOP
- Anterior segment (uveitis, cataract)
- Fundus (hemorrhage, mass)

WORK UP

Laboratory tests for patients with bilateral cataracts include:

- Calcium
- Urinalysis (urine reducing substances, amino acids)
- Chromosomes
- TORCH titers
- FTA-Abs
- Audiograms
- Electrolytes
- CBC
- Glucose
- Iron
- Galactokinase

B-scan ultrasound (by ophthalmologist) to image posterior segment and to rule out intraocular malignancy.

TREATMENT

- Referral within days
- Expedite referral if intraocular tumor suspected
- Treat systemic disease as appropriate (diabetes, electrolyte and metabolic abnormalities, infection)

TABLE 12-3 **CAUSES OF LEUKOCORIA**

Cloudy media
- Cloudy cornea
- Corneal leukoma, Peter's anomaly
- Congenital cataract
- Metabolic cataracts
- Congenital opacities
- Vitreous hemorrhage

Retinal disruption
- Retinopathy of prematurity
- Tumor (retinoblastoma)
- Intraocular infection (toxoplasmosis, toxocariasis)
- Retinal detachment
- Persistent hyperplastic primary vitreous

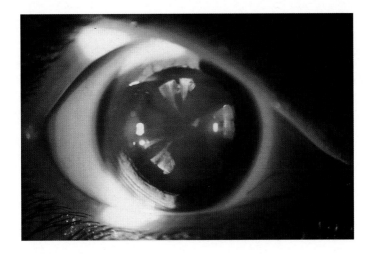

Figure 12-5 *Congenital nuclear cataract. The opacities in this case do not affect vision.*

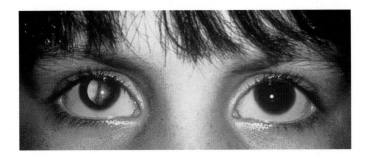

Figure 12-6 *Right leukocoria in a patient with retinoblastoma.*

FOLLOW UP

Follow up varies according to the etiology of the leukocoria.

ICD-9 CODES

360.44   Leukocoria
743.30–743.34   Congenital cataracts

NASOLACRIMAL DUCT OBSTRUCTION

HISTORY

- Tearing and excess mucus
- Redness
- Infection
- Systemic illness
- Swelling or mass
- Pulsation of mass

FINDINGS ON EXAMINATION

- Tearing (Fig. 12-7)
- Bilateral in one third of cases
- Medial canthal swelling (Fig. 12-8): above medial canthal tendon could represent a meningocele or encephalocele; below medial canthal tendon could represent a dacryocele or dacryocystitis
- Pulsation
- Discharge (mucopurulent or clear), reflux of discharge with pressure over nasolacrimal duct
- Red eye
- Crusted or matted lashes

EXAMINATION OUTLINE

- External (injection/mass/proptosis)
- Vision
- Pupils
- Motility restriction (orbital process)
- IOP
- Anterior segment
- Gentle medial canthal pressure to express material
- Dye disappearance test—instill fluorescein into conjunctival fornix and see if dye disappears
- Fundus

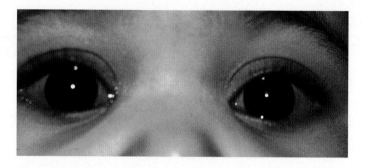

Figure 12-7 *Tearing in a patient with bilateral nasolacrimal duct obstruction. This patient does not have corneal diameters greater than 12 mm, decreasing the likelihood that the patient has congenital glaucoma.*

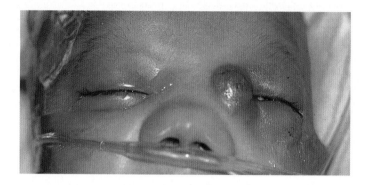

Figure 12-8 *Infected left dacryocystitis. A noninfected fluctuant mass below the medial canthal ligament is most likely a dacryocele.*

TREATMENT

- Warm compresses
- Apply finger pressure to the medial aspect of the nose near the medial canthal tendon and sweep downward over the lacrimal sac (Crigler massage); have the parent repeat 10 times each day (with each diaper change)
- Antibiotic drops are prudent if the conjunctiva is injected and/or the discharge appears purulent; may need oral or IV antibiotics if cellulitis develops
- Nonresolving cases are treated by the pediatric ophthalmologist with lacrimal duct probing, Crawford tube placement, or dacryocystorhinostomy, as the situation dictates; initial probing is successful in 90 percent

FOLLOW UP

The patient should be referred to the pediatric ophthalmologist within days. Presence of infection or other processes may dictate more expeditious referrals.

ICD-9 CODES

375.21	Epiphora due to excess lacrimation
375.22	Epiphora due to insufficient drainage
375.55	Obstruction of nasolacrimal duct, neonatal
743.65	Congenital anomaly of nasolacrimal duct

PEARLS

- If cellulitis or dacryocystitis is present, consider admission for intravenous antibiotics for infants, as dacryocystitis can quickly spread to the orbit.
- Nasolacrimal duct obstruction of the newborn occurs in 5 percent of all births.
- Majority resolve spontaneously: 60 percent resolve by 6 months, and 90 percent resolve by 9 months.
- Common ocular causes of tearing in the child may include uveitis, glaucoma, conjunctivitis, corneal abrasion, and nasolacrimal duct obstruction.
- A variety of other processes may also present as tearing and should be ruled out, especially in the newly presenting older child.

CPT CODES

68801	Dilation of lacrimal punctum
68811	Probing of nasolacrimal duct
68815	Probing of nasolacrimal duct with insertion of tube or stent

CONGENITAL GLAUCOMA

HISTORY

- Often presents with the classic triad of tearing, photophobia, and blepharospasm
- Two thirds of patients are male
- Two thirds of cases are bilateral; if detected at less than 3 months of age, the majority are bilateral
- Buphthalmos, or globe enlargement, occurs if significant glaucoma is present in a child less than 3 years of age
- Family history
- Birth history and trauma, forceps delivery

FINDINGS ON EXAMINATION

- Decreased vision
- Elevated IOP
- Pupils—may have sluggish reactivity or be mid-dilated
- Cloudy cornea (Fig. 12-9A)
- Enlarged and asymmetric corneas (Fig. 12-9B)
- Enlarged and asymmetric globe
- Epiphora—excessive tearing that runs down cheek (Fig. 12-10)

- Photophobia—extreme light sensitivity, avoids light as much as possible
- Blepharospasm
- Nystagmus
- Other ocular anomalies
- Other systemic anomalies

EXAMINATION OUTLINE

- Examine periocular area for erythema, masses, proptosis
- Check vision
- Check pupils for brisk reactivity to light
- IOP
- Anterior segment—look for irregular corneal light reflex; this may indicate corneal edema from increased intraocular pressure.
- Check fundus to determine cup to disk ratio
- Measure corneal diameter

TREATMENT

Referral for topical and systemic glaucoma medications, examination under anesthesia, surgery. Treat other systemic diseases as appropriate

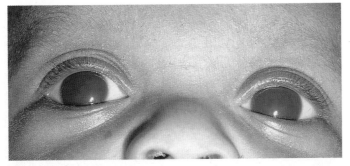

A

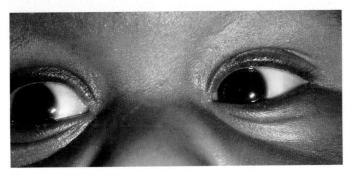

B

Figure 12-9 *A. Bilateral buphthalmos in an infant patient with congenital glaucoma. Note the cloudiness of the cornea and difficulty in discerning the pupillary margin.* ***B.*** *Twin brother with normal clear corneas.*

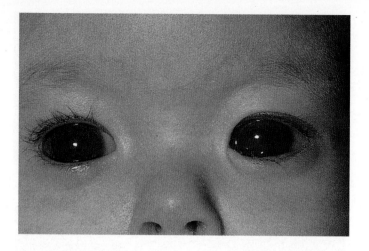

Figure 12-10 *Buphthalmos in a patient with bilateral congenital glaucoma. Note the tearing of the left eye, which can resemble naso-lacrimal duct obstruction.*

FOLLOW UP

Follow up with the pediatric ophthalmologist should occur within days, or sooner if there is infection, uveitis, or very high IOP present. Examination under anesthesia for uncooperative patients.

ICD-9 CODES

365.41   Glaucoma associated with anterior chamber angle anomalies

365.42   Glaucoma associated with anomalies of the iris

365.43   Glaucoma associated with other anterior segment anomalies

365.44   Glaucoma associated with systemic syndromes

CPT CODES

65805   Paracentesis of anterior chamber of eye with therapeutic release of aqueous

65820   Goniotomy

65850   Trabeculotomy ab externo

66180   Aqueous shunt to extraocular reservoir

PEARLS

- Early onset, corneal diameter greater than 14 mm, and afferent pupillary defects are poor prognosticators.

- The normal cup to disk ratio in children should be no greater than 0.3. Abnormal cupping can be reversible in children.

- Many other congenital ocular defects are associated with glaucoma, and are often more easily detected than the glaucoma itself.

- Surgery is the definitive cure with medical treatment providing only a temporary solution.

- Pediatric glaucoma is classified into primary congenital, secondary congenital, infantile, and juvenile types.

- Primary congenital glaucoma constitutes 50 percent of congenital glau-

coma, is idiopathic, and is present at birth.

- Secondary congenital glaucoma is due to a variety of other ocular defects and often may have systemic associations.

- Infantile glaucoma is any glaucoma with onset less than 3 years of age. The terms congenital glaucoma and infantile glaucoma are often interchanged. As with congenital glaucoma, there are primary idiopathic and secondary varieties.

- Juvenile glaucoma is pediatric glaucoma with onset greater than 3 years. It has recessive inheritance with variable penetrance and expressivity. The anatomic implication of juvenile-onset glaucoma is that the cornea and sclera have achieved sufficient structural integrity to prevent buphthalmos.

SHAKEN BABY SYNDROME

HISTORY

- Age usually less than 1 year old and always less than 3 years old
- Nature of injury (story given by caretakers often inconsistent with injury)
- Demographics: any socioeconomic class
- Acute or chronic injuries, multiple injuries in various states of healing; rib fractures are rare in accidental trauma or cardiopulmonary resuscitation
- More often bilateral, but can be unilateral
- Unwell baby: baby who cries a lot; failure to thrive; poor feeding and generally unwell
- Seizures (from brain injury)
- Recent CPR
- Birth history
- Trauma
- Hired caretakers

FINDINGS ON EXAMINATION

- Retinal hemorrhage involved: usually extensive, near macula, all layers, resolves weeks to months (Fig. 12-11)
- Vitreous hemorrhage, resolves in months to years
- Retinal folds
- Usually no cataract, no abrasion, no ocular contusion
- Various neurologic injuries: cerebral edema, hemorrhage, contusion, atrophy, subarachnoid hemorrhage, seizure activity, bradycardia, apnea, hypothermia, lethargy, and bulging fontanels
- Broken ribs
- Skin bruises

EXAMINATION OUTLINE

- Consultation of pediatrician regarding systemic findings [MRI, skeletal survey, labs (coagulation studies)]
- External (note bruising)
- Vision (often difficult in these situations and age group)
- Pupils (may be sluggish, look for APD)

- Visual fields
- Motility
- IOP
- Anterior segment (check for anterior segment injuries, hyphema)
- Fundus (retinal hemorrhages, detachment, vitreous hemorrhage)

TREATMENT

- Life support—patients often in ICU
- Treat systemic injuries
- Refer for possible vitreoretinal surgery

FOLLOW UP

In suspected cases of shaken baby syndrome, baby should be admitted to the hospital and reported to the appropriate authorities.

PEARLS

- Shaken baby syndrome occurs when the exasperated caretaker shakes the inconsolable, crying child. The acceleration–deceleration g forces exerted on the infant head causes engorgement and rupture of delicate cerebral and ocular blood vessels, inducing a characteristic pattern of brain injury.

- Accidental and birth trauma, Purtscher's syndrome, and Terson's syndrome rarely cause such extensive retinal hemorrhages, and are easily ruled out by history.

- Mortality is high, and visual prognosis is guarded.

- The retinal and vitreous hemorrhage seen in shaken baby syndrome is pathognomonic for this condition and is virtually never seen in other types of metabolic disease or nonaccidental trauma, including motor vehicle accidents and cardiopulmonary resuscitation.

ICD-9 CODE

995.55   Shaken infant syndrome

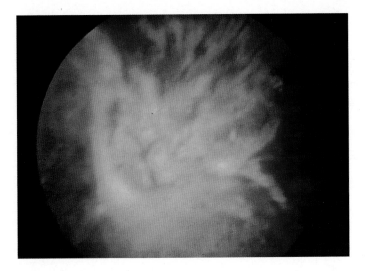

Figure 12-11 *The preretinal, subretinal, and intraretinal hemorrhages in shaken baby syndrome are usually extensive. (Courtesy of Lois Smith, MD, Boston Children's Hospital.)*

APPENDICES

SCOTT M. DAMRAUER

SUDHIR R. VORA

APPENDIX A   AMSLER GRID

PURPOSE: The Amsler Grid (Fig. A-1) is a tool for monitoring the central visual field. Distortions of the central visual field are detected by changes in the grid. Causes for central field changes include macular degeneration, macular holes, and macular edema.

METHOD   Patients with macular pathology should be given an Amsler grid to monitor changes at home. Directions for the patient:

1. Sit in an area with good lighting and hold the chart at eye level at a distance of about 14 in.

2. Wear your glasses and cover one eye.
3. With the uncovered eye, concentrate on the central dot on the grid.
4. Ask yourself the following questions as you check each eye:

   - Are any of the lines bent or crooked?
   - Are any of the boxes different in size or shape from the others?
   - Are any of the lines wavy, missing, blurry, or discolored?

If the answer to any of these questions is "yes" this may indicate that there is a change in the macula causing the distortion. The ophthalmologist can dilate the pupil and look at the macula to determine the cause.

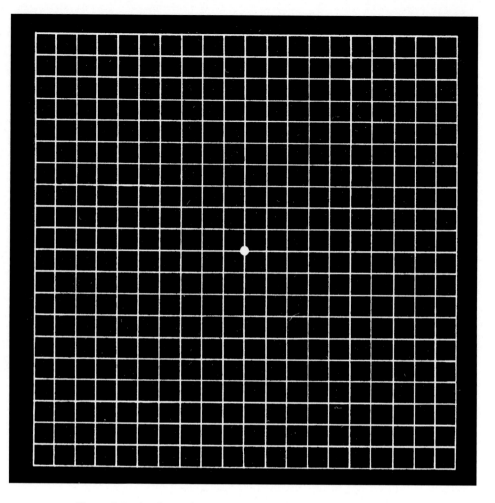

Figure A-1 *Amsler grid. Variations of the grid are possible, such as a black grid on a white background or a red grid on a black background.*

APPENDIX B   SEIDEL TEST

PURPOSE   The Seidel test is used to detect leakage of aqueous humor from the eye. Minute leakage can be seen as the dilution of dark fluorescein dye.

METHOD   While observing the eye through the slit lamp with cobalt blue light, apply fluorescein dye using a moistened fluorescein strip to the suspect area. Concentrated fluorescein does not fluoresce and appears dark orange, whereas the dilute fluorescein dye fluoresces bright green under cobalt blue light. If a leak is present, the outflow of aqueous will dilute the concentrated dye and reveal a brightly fluorescent green stream of fluid, (Fig. B-1).

A negative Seidel test does not rule out a full thickness corneal laceration. This only indicates that aqueous fluid did not exit the wound at the time of observation.

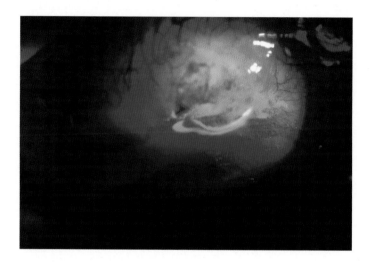

Figure B-1   *The light green stream of leaking aqueous humor is present at the superior limbus of this patient with a wound leak following cataract surgery*

APPENDIX C   OPHTHALMIC MEDICATIONS

Class	Generic Name	Trade Name*	Side Effects
Antiglaucoma			
Beta blockers	Betaxolol	Betoptic	Exacerbation of asthma,
	Carteolol	Ocupress	bradycardia, fatigue, impo-
	Levobunolol	Betagan	tence, blunting of hypo-
	Metipranolol	Optipranolol	glycemia in diabetic patient
	Timolol	Timoptic	
Alpha$_2$-selective agonists	Apraclonidine	Iopidine	Allergy
	Brimonidine	Alphagan	Tachyphylaxis
Carbonic anhydrase inhibitors	Acetazolamide	Diamox	Tingling in fingers and toes, dysgeusia, fatigue, GI upset
	Dichlorphenamide	Daranide	
	Methazolamide	Neptazane	
	Dorzolamide	Trusopt	Metallic taste
	Brinzolamide	Azopt	
Osmotics	Glycerin		Exacerbation of CHF, fluid
	Isosorbide		shifts
	Mannitol		
	Urea		
Prostaglandin analogues	Latanoprost	Xalatan	Darkening of iris color
	Travoprost	Travatan	Exacerbation of uveitis
Prostamide	Bimatoprost	Lumigan	
Docosanoid	Unoprostone	Rescula	
Sympathomimetics	Epinephrine		Adrenochrome deposits, allergy
	Dipivefrin	Propine	Epinephrine prodrug, allergy
Direct-acting cholinergic agents	Carbachol		Brow ache, retinal detach- ment, cataract formation
	Pilocarpine		
Indirect-acting cholinergic agents	Demecarium		Brow ache, retinal detach- ment, cataract formation
	Echothiophate	Phospholine iodide	
	Isofluorphate		
	Physostigmine	Eserine	

Class	Generic Name	Trade Name*	Side Effects
Antibiotics			
Sulfonamides	Sulfacetamide Trimethoprim– sulfamethox- azole		Allergy
Fluoroquinolone	Ciprofloxacin	Cipro, Ciloxan	Precipitation of drug on epithelial surface
	Norfloxacin		
	Ofloxacin	Ocuflox	
	Levofloxacin	Quixin	
Aminoglycoside	Amikacin Gentamicin Tobramycin		Epithelial toxicity
Cell-wall active	Vancomycin		
Macrolide	Erythromycin		
	Azithromycin	Zithromax	
Tetracyclines	Tetracycline Doxycycline Minocycline		
Miscellaneous	Chloramphenicol Bacitracin Clindamycin Polymyxin B		Aplastic anemia
Antifungals			
Polyene	Amphotericin B		Renal toxicity with IV dosing
	Natamycin	Natacyn	
Pyrimidine	Flucytosine		
Imidazole	Ketoconazole Miconazole Clotrimazole		
Triazole	Fluconazole		
Antivirals			
Nucleoside analogue	Trifluridine	Viroptic	
	Vidarabine	Vira-A	
	Acyclovir	Zovirax	
	Foscarnet Ganciclovir Cidofovir		

Class	Generic Name	Trade Name*	Side Effects
Anti-inflammatory			
Corticosteroids (topical)	Dexamethasone		Cataract formation
	Fluorometholone	FML	Steroid-induced glaucoma
	Medrysone	HMS	
	Loteprednol	Lotemax, Alrex	
	Prednisolone acetate		
	Prednisolone phosphate		
	Rimexolone	Alrex	
Corticosteroids (injectable)	Dexamethasone		Shortest duration
	Betamethasone		
	Triamcinolone		Deposteroid
Non steroidal anti-inflammatory medication	Ketorolac	Acular	
	Diclofenac	Voltaren	
	Flurbiprofen	Ocufen	
	Suprofen		
Anti-allergy			
Mast cell stabilizers	Cromolyn sodium	Crolom	
	Lodoxamide	Alomide	
	Pemirolast	Alamast	
Antihistamine	Levocabastine	Livostin	
	Naphazoline	Naphcon, Vasocon	
	Emedastine	Emadine	
Multiple mechanism	Olopatadine	Patanol	
	Nedocromil	Alocril	
	Ketotifen	Zaditor	
Mydriatics and Cycloplegics			
Alpha-adrenergic agonist	Phenylephrine		Hypertension with 10% solution
Parasympatholytics	Atropine		Anticholinergic toxicity
	Scopolamine		
	Homatropine		
	Cyclopentolate	Cyclogyl	
	Tropicamide	Mydriacyl	
Alpha-adrenergic blocker	Dapiprazole	Rev-Eyes	

Class	Generic Name	Trade Name*	Side Effects
Anesthetics			
	Proparacaine	Alcaine	Epithelial toxicity
	Tetracaine		
	Cocaine		Most epithelial toxic
Miscellaneous			
Hypertonic agents	Glucose		
	Hypertonic saline		
	Glycerin		

*Many of these medications are available as generics or multiple brand name products are available.

APPENDIX D   COMMON OPHTHALMIC ABBREVIATIONS AND ACRONYMS

Abbreviation	Meaning
5-FU	5-Fluorouracil
A/C	Anterior chamber
ACIOL	Anterior chamber intraocular lens
AK	Astigmatic keratotomy
ALT	Argon laser trabeculoplasty
APD, RAPD	Relative afferent pupillary defect
AR	Autorefractor measurement
ARMD	Age-related macular degeneration
BGDR	Background diabetic retinopathy
BRAO	Branch retinal artery occlusion
BRVO	Branch retinal vein occlusion
BSCL	Bandage soft contact lens
C&N	Cyclogyl and neosynephrine (dilating drops)
CF	Counting fingers
CME	Cystoid macular edema
CR	Cycloplegic refraction
CRAO	Central retinal artery occlusion
CRVO	Central retinal vein occlusion
CSME	Clinically significant macular edema
DFE	Dilated fundus examination
DR	Diabetic retinopathy
ECCE	Extracapsular cataract extraction
EKC	Epidemic keratoconjunctivitis
EOM	Extraocular muscles or motility
ET	Esotropia
FAZ	Foveal avascular zone
Gonio	Gonioscopy (examination of the angle structures of the eye)
GP-HCL	Gas permeable hard contact lens
gtt	Drop
GVF	Goldmann visual field
HM	Hand motion
HVF	Humphrey automated visual field

Abbreviation	Meaning
ICCE	Intracapsular cataract extraction
ICG	Indocyanine green dye
IK	Interstitial keratitis
IOL	Intraocular lens
IOP	Intraocular pressure
IRMA	Intraretinal microvascular abnormalities
IVFA	Intravenous fluorescein angiography
K	Cornea
KP	Keratic precipitates
L/L/L	Lids/lashes/lacrimal
LASIK	Laser-assisted in situ keratomilieusis
LLL, RLL, LUL, RUL	Left lower lid, right lower lid, etc.
LP	Light perception
LPI	Laser peripheral iridectomy
M	Manifest refraction
M&N	Mydriacyl and neosynephrine (dilating drops)
MB	Muscle balance
MCE	Microcystic corneal edema
MMC	Mitomycin C
MR	Manifest refraction
MRD	Margin-reflex distance
NLD	Nasolacrimal duct
NLP	No light perception
NS	Nuclear sclerotic cataract
NV	Near vision
NVA, NVD, NVE, NVI	Neovascularization of the angle, disk, elsewhere, iris
OAG	Open angle glaucoma
OD	Right eye
OHTN	Ocular hypertension
ON	Optic nerve
Ortho	Orthotropic
OS	Left eye
OU	Both eyes
PAS	Peripheral anterior synechiae
PBK	Pseudophakic bullous keratopathy
PCIOL	Posterior chamber intraocular lens
PCO	Posterior capsular opacification
PDR	Proliferative diabetic retinopathy
PEE	Punctate epithelial erosions

Abbreviation	Meaning
PEK	Punctate epithlial keratopathy
PH	Pinhole
Phaco	Phacoemulsification
PI	Peripheral iridectomy
PK, PKP	Penetrating keratoplasty, corneal transplant
POAG	Primary open angle glaucoma
POHS	Presumed ocular histoplasmosis syndrome
PPVx	Posterior pole vitrectomy
PRK	Photorefractive keratectomy
PRP	Panretinal photocoagultion
PSC	Posterior subcapsular cataract
PVD	Posterior vitreous detachment
PVR	Proliferative vitreoretinopathy
PXE	Pseudoexfoliation syndrome
R	Retinoscopic refraction
R/R	Recess/resect (muscle surgery)
RD	Retinal detachment
RK	Radial keratotomy
ROP	Retinopathy of prematurity
RP	Retinitis pigmentosa
RPE	Retinal pigment epithelium
Rx	Prescription
SCL	Soft contact lens
SEI	Subepithelial infiltrates (in cornea)
SLE	Slit lamp examination
SPK	Superficial punctate keratopathy
Ta	Applanation pressure
TM	Trabecular meshwork
ung	Ointment
Va	Vision
VF	Visual field
VH	Vitreous hemorrhage
Vx	Vitrectomy
W	Wearing (current glasses prescription)
XT	Exotropia
YAG	Nd:YAG laser

INDEX

Note: Page numbers followed by an italic *f* or *t* denote figures or tables, respectively.

A

Abbreviations, 267–269
Abduction, 13*t*
Abrasion, corneal, 46–49
   with chemical injury, 55, 57*f*
   examination findings, 46, 47*f*–48*f*
   examination outline, 49
   follow up, 49
   history, 46
   ICD-9 codes for, 49
   treatment, 49
Abuse, shaken baby syndrome
    with, 254
Acanthamoeba infection, 99*f*, 101
Accommodation, 8
   assessment of, 23
Acetaminophen, for hyphema, 59
Acetazolamide, 263
   for angle closure glaucoma, 137
   for central/branch retinal artery occlu-
    sion, 175
   contraindicated, in sickle cell
    patients, 61
   for neovascular glaucoma, 148
   for phacolytic glaucoma, 147
   for pseudotumor cerebri, 224
Acid injury, 55*t*, 55–58
Acyclovir, 264
   for varicella zoster virus infection, 108

Adduction, 13*t*
Adnexa, 1–4, 3*f*
Adrenergic agonist, alpha, 265
Adrenergic blocker(s)
   alpha, 265
   beta. *See* Beta blockers
Afferent pupillary defect, 233
   examination findings, 233
   examination outline, 233
   follow up, 233
   history, 233
   ICD-9 code for, 233
   treatment, 233
Age-related macular degeneration,
    180–182
   examination findings, 180, 181*f*
   examination outline, 182
   exudative (wet), 180, 181*f*
   follow up, 182
   history, 180
   ICD-9 codes for, 182
   nonexudative (dry), 180, 181*f*
Alkali injury, 45, 55–58, 55*t*, 56*f*
Allergic conjunctivitis, 92–94
   examination findings, 92, 93*f*
   examination outline, 92
   follow up, 94
   history, 92
   ICD-9 codes for, 94
   treatment, 94

Allergy medications, 265
Alpha-adrenergic agonist, 265
  alpha₂-selective, for glaucoma, 263
Alpha-adrenergic blocker, 265
Alphagan. *See* Brimonidine
Alternate cover testing, 238*t*
Amaurosis fugax
  with central/branch retinal artery occlu-
    sion, 173
  with central/branch retinal vein occlu-
    sion, 176
Amikacin, 264
  for bleb-associated infections, 144
Aminocaproic acid, for hyphema, 61
Aminoglycosides, 264
Amitriptyline, for migraine headache
    prophylaxis, 235
Amoxicillin-clavulanic acid
  for dacryocystitis, 204
  for orbital cellulitis, 195
Amphotericin B, 264
Amsler grid testing, 258, 259*f*
  in central/branch retinal vein occlusion,
    176, 178
  in macular holes, 183
  in retinal detachment, 165
Amyloidosis, systemic primary, 155
Anatomy, 1–12, 2*f*
Anesthetics, 265
Angiography, in central/branch retinal
    vein occlusion, 178
Angle closure glaucoma, 135–137
  examination findings, 135, 136*f*
  examination outline, 135
  follow up, 137
  history, 135
  ICD-9 and CPT codes for, 137
  treatment, 137
Anisocoria, 231
  examination findings, 231
  examination outline, 231, 231*f*
  follow up, 232
  history, 231
  ICD-9 codes for, 232
  treatment, 232

Annulus of Zinn, 12
Anterior chamber, 1, 2*f*
  anatomy of, 8, 9*f*
  blood/red blood cells in.
    See Hyphema
  inflammation, with endophthalmitis,
    124, 126*f*–127*f*
  slit lamp examination of, 30, 31*f*
  white blood cells in. *See* Hypopyon
Anterior chamber paracentesis, 175
Anterior ischemic optic neuropathy, 226
  examination findings, 226
  examination outline, 226
  follow up, 226
  history, 226
  ICD-9 codes for, 226
  treatment, 226
  types of, 226
Anterior segment, 1
  anatomy of, 6–8
Antibiotic(s), 264
  for bacterial conjunctivitis, 87
  for bleb-associated infections, 144
  for conjunctival/corneal
    laceration, 52
  for contact lens keratitis and
    infection, 105
  for corneal abrasion, 49
  for corneal foreign body injury, 45
  for corneal infections, 101
  for dacryocystitis, 204
  for endophthalmitis, 124
  for eyelid laceration, 79*t*
  for herpetic keratitis, 108
  for intraocular foreign body, 65
  for nasolacrimal duct obstruction, 246
  for orbital cellulitis, 195
  for traumatic glaucoma, 140
Anticoagulants, contraindicated, for
    blow-out fractures, 84
Antiemetics
  for intraocular foreign body, 65
  for ruptured globe and scleral rup-
    ture, 72
Antifungal medications, 264

Antihistamine(s), 265
  for allergic conjunctivitis, 94
  for contact dermatitis, 187
  for viral conjunctivitis, 91
Anti-inflammatory medications, 265
Antiviral medications, 264
Applanation tonometry, 32, 33*f*
Apraclonidine, 263
  for angle closure glaucoma, 137
  for phacolytic glaucoma, 147
Aqueous humor, 6, 8
Arachnoid, 2*f*
Arcuate defects, 217*t*
Arteriovenous malformation, proptosis
    with, 208
Arteritic anterior ischemic optic neuro-
    pathy, 226
Arteritis
  giant cell
    age-related macular degeneration
      with, 182
    central/branch retinal artery occlu-
      sion with, 175
    central/branch retinal vein occlusion
      with, 178
  temporal
    anterior ischemic optic neuropathy
      with, 226
    central/branch retinal artery occlu-
      sion with, 173–175
Artificial tears
  for allergic conjunctivitis, 94
  for dry eyes, 117
  for exposure keratopathy, 112
  for proptosis, 206
  for subconjunctival hemor-
    rhage, 95
  for viral conjunctivitis, 91
Aspirin
  contraindicated
    for blow-out fractures, 84
    for hyphema, 59
    for traumatic glaucoma, 140
  for migraine headache, 235
Asteroid hyalosis, 155, 156*f*

Atropine, 265
  for hyphema, 59
Augmentin. *See* Amoxicillin-
    clavulanic acid
Autoimmune disease, scleritis
    with, 122
Azithromycin, 264
Azopt. *See* Brinzolamide

B

Bacitracin, 264
Bacitracin-erythromycin, for bacterial
    conjunctivitis, 87
Bacterial conjunctivitis, 85–87
  acute, 85, 87
  chronic, 85, 87
  examination findings, 85, 86*f*
  examination outline, 87
  follow up, 87
  history, 85
  hyperacute, 85, 86*f*, 87
  ICD-9 codes for, 87
  treatment, 87
Basal cell carcinoma, 198,
    199*f*, 203
Basic ophthalmic examination,
    15–41
Bell's palsy, exposure keratopathy with,
    110–112
Bell's reflex, testing for, 110*t*
Beta blockers
  for glaucoma, 148, 152, 263
  for migraine headache prophyl-
    axis, 235
  for pseudoexfoliation syndrome, 150
Betamethasone, 265
Betaxolol, 263
Bimatoprost, 263
Binasal field defect, 217*t*, 217*f*
Binocular double vision, 218
Bitemporal hemianopia, 22*f*, 216*f*, 217*t*
Bleb-associated infections, 142–144
  examination findings, 142, 143*f*

Bleb-associated infections (*Cont.*):
  examination outline, 142
  follow up, 144
  grading of, 142*t*
  history, 142
  ICD-9 codes for, 144
  treatment, 144
Blepharitis, 113*t*, 117
Blepharospasm, with congenital glaucoma, 250
Blind spots
  enlargement of, 216*t*
  normal, 22*f*, 216*f*
Blow-out fractures, 81–84
  computed tomography of, 81,
    82*f*–83*f*
  definition of, 81
  enophthalmos of opposing eye after
    (pseudoproptosis), 208
  examination findings, 81, 82*f*
  examination outline, 81
  follow up, 84
  history, 81
  ICD-9 codes for, 84
  treatment, 84
Bowman's layer, 6, 7*f*, 9*f*
Branch retinal artery occlusion,
  173–175
  examination findings, 173, 174*f*
  examination outline, 175
  follow up, 175
  history, 173
  ICD-9 and CPT codes for, 175
  treatment, 175
Branch retinal vein occlusion,
  176–178
  examination findings, 176, 177*f*
  examination outline, 178
  follow up, 178
  history, 176
  ICD-9 codes for, 178
  imaging studies in, 178
  laboratory studies in, 178
  treatment, 178
  work up, 178

Brimonidine, 263
  for angle closure glaucoma, 137
  for hyphema, 61
  for neovascular glaucoma, 148
  for phacolytic glaucoma, 147
  for pigmentary glaucoma, 152
  for pseudoexfoliation syndrome, 150
Brinzolamide, 263
  contraindicated, in sickle cell pa-
    tients, 61
Bruckner test, 240*t*
Bulbar conjunctiva, 6
Bullous retinal detachment, 162, 163*f*
Buphthalmos, with congenital glaucoma,
  250–253, 251*f*–252*f*

C

Calcium channel blocker, for migraine
  headache prophylaxis, 235
Canaliculi, 4, 5*f*
Canal of Schlemm, 2*f*, 8, 9*f*
Cancer, skin, 198–203
Capsular deposits, with cataracts,
  130*t*, 134*f*
Carbachol, 263
Carbogen inhalation therapy, for
  central/branch retinal artery occlusion, 175
Carbonic anhydrase inhibitors
  contraindicated, in sickle cell pa-
    tients, 61
  for glaucoma, 263
Carotid-cavernous sinus fistula,
  210–212
  examination findings, 210,
    211*f*, 213*f*
  examination outline, 212
  history, 210
  ICD-9 codes for, 212
  proptosis with, 208, 212
  treatment, 212
Carteolol, 263
Caruncle, 1

Cataract(s)
  common causes of, 130*t*
  congenital, leukocoria (white pupil)
    with, 243, 245*f*
  definition of, 129
  examination findings, 129, 131*f*, 134*f*
  formation, 129
  history, 129
  ICD-9 codes for, 129
  with lens subluxation or dis-
    location, 62
  mature, 129, 130*t*, 132*f*
  ocular examination, 129
  surgery, 129, 133*f*
  treatment, 129
Cefaclor
  for dacryocystitis, 204
  for orbital cellulitis, 195
Cefalexin, for dacryocystitis, 204
Cefazolin
  for bleb-associated infections, 144
  for endophthalmitis, 124
Ceftazidime, for intraocular foreign
  body, 65
Ceftriaxone
  for bacterial conjunctivitis, 87
  for orbital cellulitis, 195
Cefuroxime, for dacryocystitis, 204
Cellulitis
  orbital, 192–195
    in diabetic patients, 172
    examination findings, 192, 193*f*
    examination outline, 192, 194*f*
    follow up, 195
    history, 192
    ICD-9 and CPT codes for, 195
    proptosis with, 192, 193*f*, 208
    treatment, 195
  preseptal, 190
    definition of, 190
    examination findings, 190, 191*f*
    examination outline, 190
    follow up, 190
    history, 190
    ICD-9 and CPT codes for, 190

Cellulitis. preseptal (*Cont.*):
    infecting organisms, 190
    treatment, 190
Cell-wall active antibiotics, 264
Central retinal artery, 2*f*
Central retinal artery occlusion, 173–175
  examination findings, 173, 174*f*
  examination outline, 175
  follow up, 175
  history, 173
  ICD-9 and CPT codes for, 175
  treatment, 175
Central retinal vein, 2*f*
Central retinal vein occlusion, 176–178
  examination findings, 176, 177*f*
  examination outline, 178
  follow up, 178
  history, 176
  ICD-9 codes for, 178
  imaging studies in, 178, 179*f*
  laboratory studies in, 178
  treatment, 178
  work up, 178
Central scotoma, 216*t*
Cephalexin
  for blow-out fractures, 84
  for eyelid laceration, 79*t*
Chalazion, 196
  definition of, 196
  examination findings, 196, 197*f*
  examination outline, 196
  history, 196
  ICD-9 and CPT codes for, 196
  treatment, 196
Chemical injury, 55–58
  components of common sources, 55*t*
  examination findings, 55, 56*f*–57*f*
  follow up, 58
  history, 55
  ICD-9 codes for, 58
  treatment, 58
Chemosis
  with allergic conjunctivitis, 92, 93*f*
  conjunctival, with chemical injury,
    55, 56*f*

Chest radiograph, in central/branch retinal vein occlusion, 178

Chiasmal lesion, 22*f*, 216*f*, 217*t*

Child abuse, shaken baby syndrome with, 254

Chlamydial inclusion conjunctivitis, 87

Chloramphenicol, 264

Cholesterosis bulbi, 155

Cholinergic agents, for glaucoma, 263

Choroid, 1, 2*f*, 12
 reddish, in retinal detachment, 162, 163*f*

Choroidal rupture, 72, 73*f*–74*f*

Cidofovir, 264

Ciliary artery, 2*f*

Ciliary body, 2*f*, 8, 9*f*, 12

Ciliary epithelium, 9*f*

Ciliary muscle, 9*f*

Ciliary nerve, 2*f*

Ciliary process, 9*f*

Ciliary vein, 8

Ciloxan. *See* Ciprofloxacin

Ciprofloxacin, 264
 for bacterial conjunctivitis, 87
 for bleb-associated infections, 144
 for contact lens keratitis and infection, 105
 for corneal abrasion, 49
 for corneal infections, 101

Clarithromycin, for bacterial conjunctivitis, 87

Cleaning solutions, for contact lens, toxicity and hypersensitivity to, 102

Clindamycin, 264

Clotrimazole, 264

Cloudy media, leukocoria (white pupil) with, 244, 244*t*

Cobalt blue light, in corneal staining, 27

Cocaine, 265

Collagen vascular diseases, dry eyes with, 113, 116–117

Color vision testing, 40, 40*f*

Commotio retinae, 68–70

Computed tomography
 of blow-out fractures, 81, 82*f*–83*f*, 84
 of orbital cellulitis, 192, 193*f*–194*f*

Computed tomography (*Cont.*):
 of strabismus, 242
 of thyroid eye disease, 209*f*

Confrontational visual fields, 20, 216*t*

Congenital cataract, leukocoria (white pupil) with, 243, 245*f*

Congenital glaucoma, 250–253
 examination findings, 250, 251*f*–252*f*
 examination outline, 250
 follow up, 253
 history, 250
 ICD-9 and CPT codes for, 253
 primary, 253
 secondary, 253
 treatment, 250

Conjunctiva, 1, 2*f*–3*f*, 9*f*, 85–95
 anatomy of, 6
 external examination of, 27
 slit lamp examination of, 30, 31*f*
 surface, normal pH of, 58

Conjunctival laceration, 50–54
 examination findings, 50–52, 51*f*, 53*f*
 examination outline, 52
 history, 50
 ICD-9 codes for, 54
 treatment, 52

Conjunctival papillae, with allergic conjunctivitis, 92, 93*f*

Conjunctivitis
 allergic, 92–94
 examination findings, 92, 93*f*
 examination outline, 92
 follow up, 94
 history, 92
 ICD-9 codes for, 94
 treatment, 94
 bacterial, 85–87
 acute, 85, 87
 chronic, 85, 87
 examination findings, 85, 86*f*
 examination outline, 87
 follow up, 87
 history, 85
 hyperacute, 85, 86*f*, 87

Conjunctivitis. bacterial (*Cont.*):
    ICD-9 codes for, 87
    treatment, 87
  chlamydial inclusion, 87
  giant papillary, 102, 104*f*
  gonococcal, 87
  viral, 88–91
    examination findings, 88, 89*f*–90*f*
    examination outline, 91
    follow up, 91
    history, 88
    ICD-9 codes for, 91
    treatment, 91
Consensual reflex, 23
Contact dermatitis, 187–189
  common ophthalmic medications
    causing, 189*t*
  examination findings, 187, 188*f*
  examination outline, 187
  follow up, 189
  ICD-9 code for, 189
  treatment, 187
Contact lens
  cleaning solutions, toxicity and hyper-
    sensitivity to, 102
  and corneal abrasions, 49
  and corneal infections, 97–101
Contact lens keratitis and infection,
    102–105
  examination findings, 102, 103*f*–
    104*f*
  examination outline, 105
  follow up, 105
  history, 102
  ICD-9 codes for, 105
  treatment, 105
Cornea, 1, 2*f,* 97–117
  anatomy of, 6, 7*f,* 9*f*
  external examination of, 27, 28*f*
  innervation of, 6
  slit lamp examination of, 30, 31*f*
Corneal abrasion, 46–49
  with chemical injury, 55, 57*f*
  examination findings, 46, 47*f*–48*f*
  examination outline, 49
  follow up, 49

Corneal abrasion (*Cont.*):
  history, 46
  ICD-9 codes for, 49
  treatment, 49
Corneal epithelial disease/problems
  with contact lens keratitis and
    infection, 102
  with herpetic keratitis, 106–108,
    107*f*
Corneal foreign body, 43–45
  examination findings, 43, 44*f*
  examination outline, 45
  follow up, 45
  history, 43
  ICD-9 and CPT codes for, 45
  surface, 43, 44*f*
  treatment, 45
Corneal infections, 97–101
  examination findings, 97, 98*f*–99*f*
  examination outline, 100
  follow up, 101
  history, 97
  ICD-9 codes for, 101
  treatment, 101
Corneal infiltrate, 43, 44*f,* 49
  with contact lens keratitis and infection,
    102
  with corneal infection, 97,
    98*f*–99*f,* 101
  subepithelial, with viral conjunctivitis,
    88, 90*f*
Corneal laceration, 50–54
  examination findings, 50–52, 51*f,* 53*f*
  examination outline, 52
  full-thickness, 52, 53*f*
  history, 50
  ICD-9 codes for, 54
  partial-thickness, 50, 51*f*
  treatment, 52
Corneal light reflex test, 238*t*
Corneal staining, 27
  in allergic conjunctivitis, 92
  in bacterial conjunctivitis, 87
  in contact lens keratitis and infection,
    105
  in corneal abrasion, 46, 47*f*

Corneal staining (*Cont.*):
  in corneal infections, 100
  in dry eyes, 114, 115*f,* 116
  in exposure keratopathy, 112
Corneal stromal disease, with herpetic
    keratitis, 106
Corneal ulcers
  with contact lens keratitis and infection,
    102
  with corneal infections
    small peripheral, 101
    vision-threatening, 101
  with exposure keratopathy, 110
Cortical spokes or wedges, with cataracts,
    129, 130*t,* 131*f*
Corticosteroids, 265. *See also* Steroid(s)
Counting fingers, for low vision testing,
    18
Cranial nerve palsy, 227–229
Cromolyn sodium, 265
Cyclopentolate, 265
  for phacolytic glaucoma, 147
  for traumatic glaucoma, 140
Cycloplegic agents, 265
  for chemical/thermal injury, 58
  for conjunctival/corneal lacerations, 52
  for contact lens keratitis and infection,
    105
  for corneal abrasion, 49
  for corneal foreign body injury, 45
  for herpetic keratitis, 108
  for hyphema, 59
  for iridocyclitis, 121
  for phacolytic glaucoma, 147
  for traumatic glaucoma, 140

D

Dacryocystitis, 204
  bacteria causing, 205*t*
  examination findings, 204, 205*f*
  examination outline, 204
  follow up, 204
  history, 204

Dacryocystitis (*Cont.*):
  ICD-9 and CPT codes for, 204
  nasolacrimal duct obstruction with,
    248*f,* 249
  treatment, 204
Dapiprazole, 265
Decongestants, for orbital cellulitis, 195
Demecarium, 263
Dendrites, with herpetic keratitis, 106–
    108, 107*f,* 109*f*
Depression (eye movement), 13*t*
Dermatitis, contact, 187–189
  common ophthalmic medications caus-
    ing, 189*t*
  examination findings, 187, 188*f*
  examination outline, 187
  follow up, 189
  ICD-9 code for, 189
  treatment, 187
Descemet's membrane, 6, 7*f,* 9*f*
  folds, with corneal infection, 97
Dexamethasone, 265
  for contact dermatitis, 187
Diabetes mellitus
  cataracts with, 129, 132*f*
  cranial nerve palsy with, 227, 229
Diabetic retinopathy, 168–172
  direct funduscopic examination in, 36
  examination findings, 168–170,
    169*f*–171*f*
  examination outline, 170
  follow up, 172
  history, 168
  ICD-9 codes for, 172
  nonproliferative, 168, 169*f*
  proliferative, 170, 171*f*
    vitreous hemorrhage with, 161
  treatment, 172
Diamox. *See* Acetazolamide
Dichlorphenamide, 263
Diclofenac, 265
Dicloxacillin, for eyelid laceration, 79*t*
Dilator muscle, of pupil, 8, 9*f*
Diphenhydramine, for contact dermatitis,
    187

Dipivefrin, 263
Diplopia (double vision), 219
    ICD-9 code for, 219
    with strabismus, 240, 242
    testing for, 218, 218*f*–219*f*
Direct funduscopic examination, 36,
        37*f*–38*f*
    in flashes and floaters, 157
    in retinal detachment, 165
    in vitreous hemorrhage, 159
Discharge
    with bacterial conjunctivitis, 85
    with corneal infections, 97, 98*f*
    with nasolacrimal duct obstruction, 246
    with viral conjunctivitis, 88
Disk hemorrhage, with angle closure glau-
        coma, 135, 136*f*
Diuretics, thiazide. *See also* Acetazolamide
    for angle closure glaucoma, 137
    for neovascular glaucoma, 148
    for phacolytic glaucoma, 147
Docosanoid, for glaucoma, 263
Dorzolamide, contraindicated, in sickle
        cell patients, 61
Double vision (diplopia), 218
    ICD-9 code for, 218
    with strabismus, 240, 242
    testing for, 219, 218*f*–219*f*
Doxycycline, 264
    for bacterial conjunctivitis, 87
Drance hemorrhage, with angle closure
        glaucoma, 135, 136*f*
Dry eyes, 113–117
    exacerbating factors, 113
    examination findings, 114, 115*f*
    examination outline, 114–116
    follow up, 117
    history, 113
    ICD-9 codes for, 117
    major causes of, 113*t*
    with rosacea, 116, 116*t*
    tear break-up time in, 116, 116*t*
    treatment, 117
Dry macular degeneration, 180, 181*f*
Dura, 2*f*

E

Echothiophate, 263
Edrophonium test, 230, 230*t*
Elevation, 13*t*
Emedastine, 265
Endophthalmitis, 124
    bleb-associated, 142*t*, 142–144
    common organisms causing, 125*t*
    follow up, 124
    history, 124
    ICD-9 and CPT codes for, 124
    laboratory work up in, 124
    ocular findings in, 124, 126*f*–127*f*
    treatment, 124
Endothelium, corneal, 6, 7*f*, 9*f*
Enophthalmos
    with blow-out fracture, 81
    of opposing eye, after blow-out frac-
        ture, 208
Epidemic keratoconjunctivitis, 89*f*
Epinephrine, 263
Epiphora, with congenital glaucoma, 250,
        252*f*
Epithelium
    ciliary, 9*f*
    corneal, 6, 7*f*, 9*f*
        in contact lens keratitis and
            infection, 102
        in herpetic keratitis, 106–108, 107*f*
        irregular, with exposure keratopathy,
            110, 111*f*
    retinal pigment, 2*f*, 10
        reddish, in retinal detachment, 162,
            163*f*
Ergotamine, for migraine headache, 235
Erythrocyte sedimentation rate
    in anterior ischemic optic neuropathy,
        226
    in central/branch retinal vein occlusion,
        178
Erythromycin, 264
    for bacterial conjunctivitis, 87
    for corneal abrasion, 49

Esotropia, 242*f*
Ethmoid bone, 12, 13*f*
Examination
  basic ophthalmic, 15–41
  color vision, 40, 40*f*
  external, 27, 28*f*–29*f*
  funduscopic, 36, 37*f*–39*f*
  motility, 26
  near vision test for, 15, 18, 19*f*
  pediatric, 237*t,* 237–238, 238*t,* 239*f*
  pupillary, 23, 24*f*–25*f*
  slit lamp, 30, 31*f*
  Snellen test for, 15, 17*f*
  stereoacuity, 41, 41*f*
  visual acuity, 15–18, 16*t,* 17*f,* 19*f*
  visual fields, 20, 21*f*–22*f*
Exophthalmos, 27
  with blow-out fracture, 81
  with central/branch retinal vein occlu-
    sion, 176
Exotropia, 242*f*
Exposure keratopathy, 110–112
  examination findings, 110, 111*f*
  examination outline, 112
  follow up, 112
  history, 110
  ICD-9 codes for, 112
  proptosis with, 206
  testing for Bell's reflex in,
    110, 110*t*
  treatment, 112
External examination, 27, 28*f*–29*f*
Extorsion, 13*t*
Extraocular muscles, 1, 12
  action of, 26*t*
  assessment of, 26
  contraction, primary direction of eye
    movement with, 13*t*
  features of, 13*t*
  innervation of, 12, 13*t,* 26*t*
Exudative macular degeneration,
    180, 181*f*
Exudative retinal detachment, 167
Eyelashes, 3*f*
  hair follicles of, 1

Eyelid(s), 1
  anatomy of, 1, 3*f*
  blood supply to, 1
  external examination of, 27, 29*f*
  innervation of, 1
  lymphatic drainage from, 1
  poor or incomplete closure of
    dry eyes with, 114, 116
    exposure keratopathy with, 110–
      112, 111*f*
  retraction, in proptosis, 206–208,
    207*f*
  retractors, 3*f*
  slit lamp examination of, 30, 31*f*
Eyelid laceration, 76–80
  examination findings, 76, 77*f*–78*f*
  examination outline, 76
  follow up, 80
  history, 76
  ICD-9 and CPT codes for, 80
  treatment, 76, 79*t*
Eyelid vesicles, herpes-related, 29*f*
Eye socket, positioning within,
  assessment of, 27

F

Finger counting, for low vision testing, 18
Flashes and floaters, 155–158
  with bacterial conjunctivitis, 85
  examination findings, 157
  examination outline, 157
  follow up, 158
  history, 155
  ICD-9 code for, 158
Fluconazole, 264
Flucytosine, 264
Fluorescein angiography, in central/branch
    retinal vein occlusion, 178
Fluorometholone, 265
Fluoroquinolone(s), 264
  for bleb-associated infections, 144
  for contact lens keratitis and infection,
    105

Flurbiprofen, 265
Focusing, 8
Foreign body
    corneal, 43–45
        examination findings, 43, 44f
        examination outline, 45
        follow up, 45
        history, 43
        ICD-9 and CPT codes for, 45
        infiltrate, 43, 44f
        surface, 43, 44f
        treatment, 45
    intraocular, 65–67
        examination findings, 65, 66f
        examination outline, 65
        history, 65
        ICD-9 and CPT codes for, 67
        treatment, 65
Foreign body sensation
    with bacterial conjunctivitis, 85
    with dry eyes, 113
    with exposure keratopathy, 110
    with viral conjunctivitis, 88
Foscarnet, 264
Fourth nerve palsy, 228
    examination findings, 228
    examination outline, 228
    follow up, 228
    history, 228
    ICD-9 code for, 228
    treatment, 228
Fovea, 10, 11f
    direct funduscopic examination of,
        36
Frontal bone, 12, 13f
Frontal sinus, 3f
Full-thickness corneal laceration, 52, 53f
Funduscopy
    direct, 36, 37f–38f
    in flashes and floaters, 157
    indirect, 39f
    pediatric, 238
    in retinal detachment, 165
    in vitreous hemorrhage, 159
Fungal disease, medications for, 264

G

Ganciclovir, 264
Gentamicin, 264
    for endophthalmitis, 124
Ghost cell glaucoma, with vitreous hem-
    orrhage, 161
Giant cell arteritis
    age-related macular degeneration with,
        182
    central/branch retinal artery occlusion
        with, 175
    central/branch retinal vein occlusion
        with, 178
Giant papillary conjunctivitis, 102, 104f
Giant retinal tear, 68–70
Gland of Krause, 3f
Gland of Wolfring, 3f
Glaucoma, 135–154
    angle closure, 135–137
        examination findings, 135, 136f
        examination outline, 135
        follow up, 137
        history, 135
        ICD-9 and CPT codes for, 137
        treatment, 137
    congenital, 250–253
        examination findings, 250, 251f–252f
        examination outline, 250
        follow up, 253
        history, 250
        ICD-9 and CPT codes for, 253
        primary, 253
        secondary, 253
        treatment, 250
    cupping, 217f
    cystoid macular edema, 217f
    direct funduscopic examination in, 36
    infantile, 253
    intraocular pressure in, measurement
        of, 32
    juvenile, 253
    medications for, 263
    pediatric, classification of, 253

Glaucoma (*Cont.*):
  phacolytic, 145–147
    examination findings, 145, 146*f*
    examination outline, 145
    follow up, 147
    history, 145
    ICD-9 codes for, 147
    treatment, 147
  pigmentary, 152
    examination findings, 152, 153*f*
    follow up, 152
    history, 152
    ICD-9 code for, 152
    treatment, 152
  secondary or ghost cell, with vitreous
    hemorrhage, 161
  steroid-induced, 154
    examination findings, 154
    follow up, 154
    history, 154
    ICD-9 code for, 154
    treatment, 154
  traumatic, 138–141
    admission for, 140
    examination findings, 138, 139*f*
    examination outline, 140
    follow up, 140
    grading of hyphema with, 138*t*
    ICD-9 code for, 140
    treatment, 140
    urgent referral for, 140
  visual field defects with, 218*t*
Glaucoma bleb, infections associated
    with, 142–144
  examination findings, 142, 143*f*
  examination outline, 142
  follow up, 144
  grading of, 142*t*
  history, 142
  ICD-9 codes for, 144
  treatment, 144
Glucose, 265
Glycerin, 263, 265
  for angle closure glaucoma, 137
Goldmann tonometer, 33*f*
Goldmann visual field, 20, 216*t*

Gonococcal conjunctivitis, 87
Gradenigo's syndrome, 229
Greater wing of sphenoid, 13*f*, 14*t*

H

Hand motion testing, 18
Headache, migraine, 234–235
  classification of, 234*t*
  examination findings, 234
  examination outline, 234
  follow up, 235
  history, 234
  ICD-9 codes for, 235
  treatment, 235
Hemianopia, 22*f*, 216*f*, 217*t*
Hemorrhage
  disk, with angle closure glaucoma, 135,
    136*f*
  Drance, with angle closure glaucoma,
    135, 136*f*
  preretinal, 68–70, 71*f*
  retinal, with shaken baby syndrome,
    254, 255*f*
  subconjunctival, 95
    with corneal infections, 97
    examination findings, 95, 96*f*
    examination outline, 95
    follow up, 95
    history, 95
    ICD-9 codes for, 95
    treatment, 95
  subconjunctival petechial, with viral
    conjunctivitis, 88, 89*f*
  vitreous, 159–161
    with diabetic retinopathy, 168, 170
    examination findings, 159, 160*f*
    examination outline, 159
    flashes and floaters with, 155–158
    follow up, 161
    history, 159
    ICD-9 code for, 161
    imaging studies in, 161
    laboratory studies in, 161
    with shaken baby syndrome, 254

Hemorrhage. vitreous (*Cont.*):
    treatment, 161
    work up in, 161
Herpes simplex virus infection
  corneal, 100
  eyelid vesicles with, 29*f*
  keratitis with, 106–108
    examination findings, 106, 107*f*
    examination outline, 108, 109*f*
    follow up, 108
    history, 106
    ICD-9 codes for, 108
    ocular signs of, 106
    skin signs of, 106
    treatment, 108
  preseptal cellulitis with, 190
Hirschberg test, 238, 240*t*
Hollenhorst plaque, 174*f*
Homatropine, 265
Homonymous hemianopia, 22*f*, 217*t*
Humidity, low, and dry eyes, 113
Humphrey visual field, 20, 217*t*, 218*f*–219*f*
Hypertonic agents, 265
Hypertonic saline, 265
Hyphema, 59–61
  concomitant signs related to trauma,
    59, 60*f*
  with corneal infections, 97
  examination findings, 59, 60*f*
  examination outline, 59
  with eyelid laceration, 76
  follow up, 61
  grading of, 139*t*
  history, 59
  ICD-9 codes for, 61
  with traumatic glaucoma, 138–141,
    139*f*
  treatment, 59–60
  with vitreous hemorrhage, 159
Hypopyon
  with bleb-association infections, 142
  with corneal infections, 97, 98*f*, 100
  with endophthalmitis, 124, 126*f*
  with herpetic keratitis, 106
  with iridocyclitis and traumatic iritis,
    119, 120*f*

Hypopyon (*Cont.*):
  with tight contact lens syndrome, 102
  with viral conjunctivitis, 88

I

Ibuprofen, for migraine headache, 235
Imidazole, 264
Indirect funduscopic examination, 39*f*
Indomethacin, for scleritis, 122
Infantile glaucoma, 253
Infection(s)
  bleb-associated, 142–144
    examination findings, 142, 143*f*
    examination outline, 142
    follow up, 144
    grading of, 142*t*
    history, 142
    ICD-9 codes for, 144
    treatment, 144
  contact lens-associated, 102–105
    examination findings, 102,
      103*f*–104*f*
    examination outline, 105
    follow up, 105
    history, 102
    ICD-9 codes for, 105
    treatment, 105
  corneal, 97–101
    examination findings, 97, 98*f*–99*f*
    examination outline, 100
    follow up, 101
    history, 97
    ICD-9 codes for, 101
    treatment, 101
  herpes simplex virus. *See* Herpes simplex virus infection
  varicella zoster virus. *See* Varicella zoster virus infection
Inferior oblique muscle, 3*f*, 12
  action of, 26*t*
  assessment of, 26
  contraction, primary direction of eye
    movement with, 13*t*
  innervation of, 13*t*

Inferior orbital fissure, 13*f*, 14*t*
Inferior rectus muscle, 12
  action of, 26*t*
  assessment of, 26
  contraction, primary direction of eye
    movement with, 13*t*
  innervation of, 13*t*
Infraorbital foramen, 13*f*
Infraorbital groove, 13*f*
Insulin therapy, and diabetic retinopathy, 172
Intorsion, 13*t*
Intraocular foreign body, 65–67
  examination findings, 65, 66*f*
  examination outline, 65
  history, 65
  ICD-9 and CPT codes for, 67
  treatment, 65
Intraocular pressure
  abnormal values of, 32
  in bleb-associated infections, 142
  in central/branch retinal artery occlu-
    sion, 175
  elevated
    with angle closure glaucoma, 135–
     137
    with carotid-cavernous sinus
     fistula, 212
    with hyphema, 59–61
    with iridocyclitis, 121
    with neovascular glaucoma, 148
    with phacolytic glaucoma, 145–147
    with pigmentary glaucoma, 152
    with steroid-induced glaucoma,
     154
    with traumatic glaucoma, 138–141
  with flashes and floaters, 157
  measurement of, 32–34
    applanation tonometry for, 32, 33*f*
    manual assessment for, 34
    pediatric, 237
    Schiotz tonometry for, 34, 35*f*
  normal values of, 32
  in pseudoexfoliation syndrome, 150
  in retinal detachment, 165
  in vitreous hemorrhage, 159, 161

Intraretinal microvascular abnormalities,
  with nonproliferative diabetic
  retinopathy, 168
IOP. *See* Intraocular pressure
Iopidine. *See* Apraclonidine
Iridocyclitis, 119–121
  common causes of, 121*t*
  examination outline, 119
  follow up, 121
  history, 119
  ICD-9 codes for, 121
  laboratory work up in, 119
  ocular findings, 119, 120*f*
  treatment, 121
Iridodonesis, with lens subluxation or
  dislocation, 62
Iris, 1, 2*f*, 12
  anatomy of, 8, 9*f*
  slit lamp examination of, 30,
    31*f*
Iritis
  with herpetic keratitis, 106
  traumatic, 119–121
    examination outline, 119
    follow up, 121
    history, 119
    ICD-9 codes for, 121
    laboratory work up in, 119
    ocular findings, 119, 120*f*
    treatment, 121
Isofluorphate, 263
Isosorbide, 263
  for angle closure glaucoma, 137

J

Juvenile glaucoma, 253

K

Keratic precipitates
  with iridocyclitis and traumatic iritis,
    119, 120*f*, 121
  with phacolytic glaucoma, 145

Keratitis
    contact lens, 102–105
        examination findings, 102, 103*f*–
            104*f*
        examination outline, 105
        follow up, 105
        history, 102
        ICD-9 codes for, 105
        treatment, 105
    herpetic, 106–108
        examination findings, 106,
            107*f*
        examination outline, 108, 109*f*
        follow up, 108
        history, 106
        ICD-9 codes for, 108
        ocular signs of, 106
        skin signs of, 106
        treatment, 108
Keratoconjunctivitis, pseudosuperior lim-
    bic, 102
Keratoconjunctivitis sicca (dry eyes),
    113–117
    exacerbating factors, 113
    examination findings, 114, 115*f*
    examination outline, 114–116
    follow up, 117
    history, 113
    ICD-9 codes for, 117
    major causes of, 113*t*
    with rosacea, 116, 116*t*
    tear break-up time in, 116, 116*t*
    treatment, 117
Keratopathy, exposure, 110–112
    examination findings, 110, 111*f*
    examination outline, 112
    follow up, 112
    history, 110
    ICD-9 codes for, 112
    proptosis with, 206
    testing for Bell's reflex in, 110,
        110*t*
    treatment, 112
Ketoconazole, 264
Ketorolac, 265
Ketotifen, 265

Krimsky test, 238*t*
Krukenberg's spindle, with pigmen-
    tary glaucoma, 152, 153*f*

L

Laceration(s)
    conjunctival and corneal, 50–54
        examination findings, 50–52, 51*f*,
            53*f*
        examination outline, 52
        history, 50
        ICD-9 codes for, 54
        treatment, 52
    eyelid, 76–80
        examination findings, 76,
            77*f*–78*f*
        examination outline, 76
        follow up, 80
        history, 76
        ICD-9 and CPT codes for, 80
        treatment, 76, 79*t*
Lacrimal apparatus, 1
    anatomy of, 4, 5*f*
    blood supply to, 4
    innervation of, 4
    lymphatic drainage from, 4
Lacrimal artery, 1
Lacrimal bone, 12, 13*f*
Lacrimal gland tumors, proptosis with,
    208
Lacrimal groove, 13*f*
Lacrimal sac, 4, 5*f*
Lagophthalmos
    dry eyes with, 114, 116
    exposure keratopathy with, 110–
        112
    nocturnal, 110
    in proptosis, 206
Latanoprost, 263
    for neovascular glaucoma, 148
    for pigmentary glaucoma, 152
    for pseudoexfoliation syndrome,
        150
Lateral canthus, 1

Lateral rectus muscle, 2*f,* 12
    action of, 26*t*
    assessment of, 26
    contraction, primary direction of eye
        movement with, 13*t*
    innervation of, 13*t*
Left homonymous superior quadran-
        tanopia, 22*f,* 216*f*
Lens, 1, 129
    anatomy of, 8, 9*f*
    slit lamp examination of, 30, 31*f*
    transparency, loss of. *See* Cataract(s)
Lens capsule, 2*f*
Lens subluxation or dislocation, 62
    examination findings, 62, 63*f*–64*f*
    examination outline, 62
    follow up, 62
    history, 62
    ICD-9 code for, 62
    treatment, 62
Lesser wing of sphenoid, 13*f,* 14*t*
Leukocoria (white pupil), 244–246
    causes of, 244*t*
    examination findings, 244, 245*f*
    examination outline, 244
    follow up, 246
    history, 244
    ICD-9 codes for, 246
    imaging studies in, 244
    laboratory tests in, 244
    treatment, 244
    work up, 244
Levator palpebrae aponeurosis, 3*f*
Levator palpebrae muscle, 3*f*
Levobunolol, 263
    for central/branch retinal artery
        occlusion, 175
Levocabastine, 265
Levofloxacin, 264
    for bleb-associated infections, 144
Lids. *See* Eyelid(s)
Lightning. *See* Flashes and
        floaters
Light perception testing, 18
Limbus, 6

Lodoxamide, 265
Loteprednol, 265
Low vision testing, 18
Lubricating ointment
    for dry eyes, 117
    for proptosis, 206

M

Macrolides, 264
    for bacterial conjunctivitis, 87
Macula, 2*f,* 10
    direct funduscopic examination of,
        36
    pathology, Amsler grid testing in,
        258, 259*f*
Macular degeneration
    age-related, 180–182
        examination findings, 180, 181*f*
        examination outline, 182
        exudative (wet), 180, 181*f*
        follow up, 182
        history, 180
        ICD-9 codes for, 182
        nonexudative (dry), 180, 181*f*
    direct funduscopic examination in,
        36
Macular holes, 183–185
    examination findings, 183, 184*f*
    examination outline, 185
    follow up, 185
    history, 183
    ICD-9 code for, 185
    traumatic, 68–70, 71*f*
    treatment, 185
    Watkze-Allen test for, 185, 185*t*
Magnetic resonance imaging, in
        strabismus, 242
Malignant melanoma, 200, 202*f*
Mannitol, 263
Manual assessment, of intraocular
        pressure, 34
Marcus-Gunn pupil, 23
    with retinal detachment, 162

Marfan's syndrome, lens subluxation or dislocation with, 62, 63*f*

Mast cell stabilizers, 265

Maxilla bone, 12, 13*f*
 in blow-out fracture, 81–84

Medial canthus, 1, 4
 swelling, with nasolacrimal duct obstruction, 246, 247*f*

Medial rectus muscle, 2*f*, 12
 action of, 26*t*
 assessment of, 26
 contraction, primary direction of eye movement with, 13*t*
 innervation of, 13*t*

Medications, 263–265

Medrysone, 265

Meibomian glands, 1, 3*f*

Melanoma, malignant, 200, 202*f*

Metamorphopsia
 with central/branch retinal vein occlusion, 176, 178
 with macular holes, 183
 with retinal detachment, 162, 165

Methazolamide, contraindicated, in sickle cell patients, 61

Methylprednisolone
 for anterior ischemic optic neuropathy, 226
 for optic neuritis, 221

Metipranolol, 263

Miconazole, 264

Microhyphema, 59

Migraine headache, 234–235
 classification of, 234*t*
 examination findings, 234
 examination outline, 234
 follow up, 235
 history, 234
 ICD-9 codes for, 235
 treatment, 235

Minocycline, 264

Monocular double vision, 219

Motility examination, 26
 in blow-out fracture, 81, 82*f*
 pediatric, 238

Mucormycosis, 172, 195

Muscle(s), extraocular, 1, 12
 action of, 26*t*
 assessment of, 26
 contraction, primary direction of eye movement with, 13*t*
 features of, 13*t*
 innervation of, 12, 13*t*, 26*t*

Muscle balance testing, 238, 238*t*

Myasthenia gravis, 230
 examination outline, 230
 follow up, 230
 history, 230
 ICD-9 code for, 230
 Tensilon test for, 230, 230*t*
 treatment, 230

Mydriatics, 265

N

Nafcillin, for orbital cellulitis, 195

Naphazoline, 265
 for contact dermatitis, 187

Naphazoline/pheniramine
 for allergic conjunctivitis, 94
 for viral conjunctivitis, 91

Nasolacrimal duct obstruction (NLDO), 247–249
 examination findings, 247, 248*f*
 examination outline, 247
 follow up, 244
 history, 247
 ICD-9 and CPT codes for, 249
 treatment, 249

Nasolacrimal sac, 4, 5*f*

Natamycin, 264

Near vision test/near card, 15, 18, 19*f*

Nedocromil, 265

Neovascular glaucoma, 148
 examination findings, 148, 149*f*
 follow up, 148
 history, 148
 ICD-9 codes for, 148
 treatment, 148

Neptazane. *See* Methazolamide
Neuroophthalmology, 215–235
Neurosensory layer, of retina, 10
Neurotrophic (sterile) ulcer, with herpetic keratitis, 106
NLDO. *See* Nasolacrimal duct obstruction
Nocturnal lagophthalmos, 110
Nonarteritic anterior ischemic optic neuropathy, 226
Nonexudative macular degeneration, 180, 181*f*
Nonproliferative diabetic retinopathy, 168, 169*f*
Nonsteroidal anti-inflammatory drugs, 265
  contraindicated
    for hyphema, 59
    for traumatic glaucoma, 140
  for corneal abrasion, 49
  for scleritis, 122
Norfloxacin, 264
Nuclear sclerotic cataract, 129, 130*t*, 131*f*
Nucleoside analogues, 264
Nystagmus, assessment for, 26

O

Occipital cortex, nerve pathways from retina, 21*f*
Ocuflox. *See* Ofloxacin
OD (oculus dexter), 15
Ofloxacin, 264
  for bacterial conjunctivitis, 87
  for bleb-associated infections, 144
  for contact lens keratitis and infection, 105
  for corneal abrasion, 49
  for corneal infections, 101
  for dacryocystitis, 204
  for orbital cellulitis, 195
Olopatadine, 265
Opacities, with cataracts, 129, 130*t*, 132*f*
Ophthalmic abbreviations, 267–269

Ophthalmic artery, 1
Ophthalmic medications, 263–266
Ophthalmoscopy
  direct, 36, 37*f*–38*f*
  in flashes and floaters, 157
  indirect, 39*f*
  pediatric, 238
  in retinal detachment, 165
  in vitreous hemorrhage, 159
Optic canal, 14*t*
Optic disk, 2*f*
Optic foramen, 13*f*
Optic nerve, 2*f*, 10, 11*f*
  color vision testing of, 40, 40*f*
  damage, afferent pupillary defect with, 233
  direct funduscopic examination of, 36, 37*f*–38*f*
Optic neuritis, 220–221
  examination findings, 220
  examination outline, 220
  follow up, 221
  history, 220
  ICD-9 code for, 220
  treatment, 221
Optic neuropathy
  anterior ischemic, 226
    examination findings, 226
    examination outline, 226
    follow up, 226
    history, 226
    ICD-9 codes for, 226
    treatment, 226
    types of, 226
  traumatic, 75
    examination findings, 75
    examination outline, 75
    follow up, 75
    history, 75
    ICD-9 codes for, 75
    treatment, 75
Optic pathway, lesions, and corresponding visual field defects, 22*f*, 216*f*
Orange-peel appearance, of retinal surface, 162

Ora serrata, 9f
Orbicularis oculi muscles, 1, 3f
Orbit, 1, 187–212
    anatomy of, 12, 13f
    fossae of, 12, 14t
Orbital cellulitis, 192–195
    in diabetic patients, 172
    examination findings, 192, 193f
    examination outline, 192, 194f
    follow up, 195
    history, 192
    ICD-9 and CPT codes for, 195
    proptosis with, 192, 193f, 208
    treatment, 195
Orbital fat, 3f
Orbital inflammatory pseudotumor, 208
Orbital plate of frontal bone, 13f
Orbital septum, 3f
Orbital surface
    of maxilla bone, 13f
    of zygomatic bone, 13f
Orbital tumors, proptosis with, 208
Organic solvent injury, 55t, 55–58
OS (oculus sinister), 15
Osmotics, for glaucoma, 263

P

Palatine bone, 12
Palpebral conjunctiva, 6
Palpebral fissure, 1
Papilledema, 222, 224
    direct funduscopic examination in,
        36
    examination findings, 222, 223f
    examination outline, 222
    history, 222
    ICD-9 code for, 222
    treatment, 222
Parasympatholytics, 265
Parotid nodes, 1
Pars plana, 2f, 9f
Pars plicata, 2f
Partial-thickness corneal laceration, 50, 51f

Peau d'orange appearance, of retinal sur-
        face, 162
Pediatric ophthalmology, 237–254
    special considerations in, 237–238
PEEs. See Punctate epithelial erosions
Pemirolast, 265
Penicillin V, for eyelid laceration, 79t
Petechial hemorrhage, subconjunctival,
        with viral conjunctivitis, 88, 89f
pH
    in chemical injury, 55–58
    of conjunctival surface, normal, 58
    of tears, 4
Phacodonesis, with lens subluxation or
        dislocation, 62
Phacolytic glaucoma, 145–147
    examination findings, 145, 146f
    examination outline, 145
    follow up, 147
    history, 145
    ICD-9 codes for, 147
    treatment, 147
Pharyngoconjunctival fever, 88
Phenothiazines, cataracts induced by,
        130t, 134f
Phenylephrine, 265
Photophobia
    with allergic conjunctivitis, 92
    with bacterial conjunctivitis, 85
    with congenital glaucoma, 250
    with dry eyes, 113
    with herpetic keratitis, 108
    with viral conjunctivitis, 88
Physostigmine, 263
Pia, 2f
Pigmentary glaucoma, 152
    examination findings, 152, 153f
    follow up, 152
    history, 152
    ICD-9 code for, 152
    treatment, 152
Pilocarpine, 263
    for angle closure glaucoma, 137
    for hyphema, 61
Pinhole testing, 18

Plastics, 187–212
Plica semilunaris, 1
Pneumatic retinopexy, 166
Polyene, 264
Polymyxin-bacitracin, for corneal
    abrasion, 49
Polytrim. *See* Trimethoprim-polymixin
Posterior chamber, 2*f*
Posterior segment, 1
    anatomy of, 10–12
    funduscopic examination of, 36, 37*f*–
        38*f*
Posterior subcapsular cataract, 129, 130*t,*
    133*f*
Posterior vitreous detachment
    flashes and floaters with, 158
    retinal detachment with, 167
Preauricular nodes, 1
Prednisolone
    for iridocyclitis, 121
    for phacolytic glaucoma, 147
Prednisolone acetate, 265
    for hyphema, 59
    for traumatic glaucoma, 140
Prednisolone phosphate, 265
Prednisone
    for anterior ischemic optic neuro-
        pathy, 226
    for optic neuritis, 221
Preretinal hemorrhage, 68–70, 71*f*
Presbyopia, and Snellen test, 15
Preseptal cellulitis, 190
    definition of, 190
    examination findings, 190, 191*f*
    examination outline, 190
    follow up, 190
    history, 190
    ICD-9 and CPT codes for, 190
    infecting organisms, 190
    treatment, 190
Proliferative diabetic retinopathy, 170,
    171*f*
    vitreous hemorrhage with, 161
Propanolol, for migraine headache
    prophylaxis, 235

Proparacaine, 265
    in allergic conjunctivitis, 92
    in chemical/thermal injury, 58
    in corneal infections, 100
    in dry eyes, 114
    in exposure keratopathy, 112
    in herpetic keratitis, 108
    in subconjunctival hemorrhage, 95
    in viral conjunctivitis, 91
Proptosis, 206–208
    with carotid-cavernous sinus fistula,
        208, 212
    definition of, 206
    etiology of, 208
    examination findings, 206, 207*f*
    examination outline, 206
    follow up, 208
    history, 206
    ICD-9 and CPT codes for, 208
    with orbital cellulitis, 192, 193*f,*
        208
    with thyroid eye disease, 206–208,
        207*f,* 209*f*
    treatment, 206
Prostaglandin analogues
    for glaucoma, 263
    for hyphema, 61
Prostamide, for glaucoma, 263
Pseudoexfoliation syndrome, 150
    examination findings, 150, 151*f*
    follow up, 150
    history, 150
    ICD-9 code for, 150
    treatment, 150
Pseudoproptosis, 208
Pseudosuperior limbic keratoconjunc-
    tivitis, 102
Pseudotumor cerebri, 222, 224
    examination findings, 224,
        225*f*
    examination outline, 224
    follow up, 224
    history, 224
    ICD-9 codes for, 224
    treatment, 224

Ptosis, 27
Punctae, 4, 5*f*
Punctate epithelial erosions (PEEs)
  with contact lens keratitis and infection, 102
  with dry eyes, 116
  with exposure keratopathy, 110
Pupil(s), 2*f*
  abnormal, 230
    examination findings, 231
    examination outline, 231, 231*f*
    follow up, 232
    history, 231
    ICD-9 codes for, 232
    treatment, 232
  examination, 23, 24*f*–25*f*
    pediatric, 237
  muscles of, 8, 9*f*
  white (leukocoria), 243–244
    causes of, 244*t*
    examination findings, 243, 245*f*
    examination outline, 243
    follow up, 244
    history, 243
    ICD-9 codes for, 244
    imaging studies in, 243
    laboratory tests in, 243
    treatment, 243
    work up, 243
Pupillary defect, afferent, 233
  examination findings, 233
  examination outline, 233
  follow up, 233
  history, 233
  ICD-9 code for, 233
  treatment, 233
Pupillary reflex arc, 23
Pyrimidine, 264

Q

Quadrantanopia, 22*f*, 216*f*
Quixin (levofloxacin), 264
  for bleb-associated infections, 144

R

Ranitidine
  for anterior ischemic optic neuropathy, 226
  for optic neuritis, 221
Recurrent erosion syndrome, 50
  examination outline, 50
  history, 50
  ICD-9 codes for, 50
  treatment, 50
Red blood cells, in anterior chamber. *See* Hyphema
Red eye, differential diagnosis of, 86*t*
Retina, 1, 2*f*, 155–185
  anatomy of, 10, 11*f*
  blood supply to, 10
  color vision testing of, 40, 40*f*
  direct funduscopic examination of, 36, 37*f*–38*f*
  disruption, leukocoria (white pupil) with, 244, 244*t*
  nerve pathways to occipital cortex, 21*f*
Retinal artery
  branch, occlusion of, 173–175, 174*f*
  central, 2*f*
    occlusion of, 173–175, 174*f*
Retinal damage, traumatic, 68–70
  examination findings, 68–70, 69*f*, 71*f*
  examination outline, 70
  history, 68
  ICD-9 codes for, 70
  treatment, 70
Retinal detachment, 68–70, 69*f*, 162–167
  bullous, 162, 163*f*
  causes of, 167
  examination findings, 162, 163*f*–164*f*
  examination outline, 165
  exudative, 167
  flashes and floaters with, 155–158
  follow up, 166
  history, 162

Retinal detachment (*Cont.*):
 ICD-9 code for, 166
 inflammatory, 166
 neovascular glaucoma with, 148,
  149*f*
 prognosis, 166
 rhegmatogenous, 167
 risk factors for, 162
 surgery, 166
 traction, 167
  with diabetic retinopathy, 168
 treatment, 166
 ultrasonography of, 165
 work up in, 165
Retinal foreign body, 65–67, 66*f*
Retinal hemorrhage, with shaken baby
  syndrome, 254, 255*f*
Retinal occlusion, direct funduscopic
  examination in, 36
Retinal pigment epithelium, 2*f*, 10
 reddish, in retinal detachment, 162,
  163*f*
Retinal tear, giant, 68–70
Retinal vein
 branch, occlusion of, 176–178, 177*f*
 central, 2*f*
  occlusion of, 176–178, 177*f*,
   179*f*
Retinoblastoma, leukocoria (white pupil)
  with, 245*f*
Rhegmatogenous retinal detachment,
  167
Rheumatoid arthritis, scleritis with,
  122
Right congruous incomplete homonymous
  hemianopia, 22*f*, 216*f*
Right homonymous hemianopia, 22*f*,
  217*f*
Right homonymous inferior quadrantanopia, 22*f*, 216*f*
Right incongruous hemianopia, 22*f*,
  217*f*
Rimexolone, 265
Rosacea, 116, 116*t*
Rubeosis irides, with central/branch retinal vein occlusion, 176, 178

Ruptured globe, 72
 with conjunctival laceration, 52
 examination findings, 72, 73*f*–
  74*f*
 examination outline, 72
 with eyelid laceration, 76, 80
 follow up, 72
 history, 72
 ICD-9 codes for, 72
 treatment, 72

S

Sarcoidosis, dry eyes with, 113, 116
Scattered focal defects, 216*t*
Schiotz tonometry, 34, 35*f*
Sclera, 1, 2*f*, 9*f*, 12
Scleral buckle, 166
Scleral rupture, 72
 examination findings, 72, 73*f*–74*f*
 examination outline, 72
 follow up, 72
 history, 72
 ICD-9 codes for, 72
 with intraocular foreign body, 67
 treatment, 72
Scleral sinus, 8
Scleral spur, 9*f*
Scleritis, 122
 examination outline, 122
 follow up, 122
 history, 122
 ICD-9 code for, 122
 laboratory work up in, 122
 ocular findings, 122, 123*f*
 treatment, 122
Scopolamine, 265
 for contact lens keratitis and
  infection, 105
 for herpetic keratitis, 108
Sebaceous gland carcinoma, 200, 201*f*,
  203
Sebaceous glands of Zeis, 1
Sebum, 1
Seidel test, 261, 261*f*

Senile cataract, 129
Sensory strabismus, 242
Sexual history, and bacterial conjunc-
    tivitis, 85
Shafer's sign
    with flashes and floaters, 157
    with retinal detachment, 162,
        165
    with vitreous hemorrhage, 159
Shaken baby syndrome, 254
    examination findings, 254, 255*f*
    examination outline, 254
    follow up, 254
    history, 254
    ICD-9 code for, 254
    treatment, 254
Sickle cell patients, hyphema in, 59,
    61
Sixth nerve palsy, 229
    examination findings, 229
    examination outline, 229
    follow up, 229
    history, 229
    ICD-9 code for, 229
    treatment, 229
Skin cancers, 198–203
    biopsy, 200
    differential diagnosis, 203
    examination findings, 198–200, 199*f,*
        201*f*–202*f*
    examination outline, 200
    follow up, 203
    history, 198
    ICD-9 and CPT codes for, 203
    surgical excision, 200
    treatment, 200
Sleep apnea, and exposure keratopathy,
    110–112
Slit lamp examination, 30, 31*f*
    in allergic conjunctivitis, 92
    in bacterial conjunctivitis, 87
    in contact lens keratitis and infection,
        105
    in corneal infections, 100
    in diabetic retinopathy, 170
    in flashes and floaters, 157

Slit lamp examination (*Cont.*):
    in retinal detachment, 165
    in vitreous hemorrhage, 159
Snellen test, 15, 17*f*
Solu-Medrol. *See* Methylprednisolone
Sphenoid bone, 12, 13*f,* 14*t*
Sphincter muscle, of pupil, 8, 9*f*
Squamous cell carcinoma, 200, 201*f,*
    203
Stereoacuity
    assessment of, 41, 41*f*
    definition of, 41
Steroid(s), 265
    for central/branch retinal artery
        occlusion, 175
    for contact dermatitis, 187
    for iridocyclitis, 121
    for optic neuritis, 221
    for scleritis, 122
    for traumatic optic neuropathy,
        75
Steroid-induced glaucoma, 154
    examination findings, 154
    follow up, 154
    history, 154
    ICD-9 code for, 154
    treatment, 154
Strabismus, 241–243
    examination findings, 241, 242*f*
    examination outline, 243
    follow up, 243
    history, 241
    ICD-9 codes for, 243
    treatment, 243
Stroke, visual field defects with, 217*t,*
    218*f*–219*f*
Stroma, 6, 7*f,* 9*f*
Stromal disease, corneal, with herpetic
    keratitis, 106
Stye, 196
    definition of, 196
    examination findings, 196, 197*f*
    examination outline, 196
    history, 196
    ICD-9 and CPT codes for, 196
    treatment, 196

Subarachnoid hemorrhage, vitreous hemorrhage with, 161
Subconjunctival hemorrhage, 95
  with corneal infections, 97
  examination findings, 95, 96*f*
  examination outline, 95
  follow up, 95
  history, 95
  ICD-9 codes for, 95
  treatment, 95
Subconjunctival petechial hemorrhage, with viral conjunctivitis, 88, 89*f*
Subdural hemorrhage, vitreous hemorrhage with, 161
Subepithelial infiltrate, with contact lens keratitis and infection, 102, 103*f*
Submandibular nodes, 1
Sulfacetamide, 264
  for bacterial conjunctivitis, 87
Sulfonamides, 264
Sumatriptan, for migraine headache, 235
Superficial punctate keratitis, 92
Superior oblique muscle, 12
  action of, 26*t*
  assessment of, 26
  contraction, primary direction of eye movement with, 13*t*
  innervation of, 13*t*
Superior orbital fissure, 13*f*, 14*t*
Superior rectus muscle, 12
  action of, 26*t*
  assessment of, 26
  contraction, primary direction of eye movement with, 13*t*
  innervation of, 13*t*
Superior tarsal muscle, 3*f*
Supraorbital notch, 13*f*
Suprofen, 265
Sweat glands of Moll, 1
Swinging light test, 23, 24*f*–25*f*
Sympathomimetics, for glaucoma, 263
Systemic primary amyloidosis, 155

T

Tarsorrhaphy, for proptosis, 206
Tarsus, 1
Tear (s)
  artificial. *See* Artificial tears
  composition of, 4
  with congenital glaucoma, 250, 252*f*
  layers, thickness of, 4
  with nasolacrimal duct obstruction, 246, 247*f*
  pH of, 4
  production of, 4
    decreased, dry eyes with, 113*t*
Tear break-up time, 116, 116*t*
Tear film, unstable, dry eyes with, 113*t*, 114, 115*f*
Temporal arteritis
  anterior ischemic optic neuropathy with, 226
  central/branch retinal artery occlusion with, 173–175
Tensilon test, 230, 230*t*
Terson's syndrome, vitreous hemorrhage with, 161
Tetracaine, 265
  for chemical/thermal injury, 58
Tetracyclines, 264
  for bacterial conjunctivitis, 87
Thermal injury, 55–58
  examination findings, 55
  follow up, 58
  history, 55
  ICD-9 codes for, 58
  treatment, 58
Thiazide diuretics. *See also* Acetazolamide
  for angle closure glaucoma, 137
  for neovascular glaucoma, 148
  for phacolytic glaucoma, 147
Third nerve palsy, 227
  examination findings, 227
  examination outline, 227
  follow up, 227

Third nerve palsy (*Cont.*):
  history, 227
  ICD-9 codes for, 227
  treatment, 227
Thyroid eye disease, proptosis with,
  206–208, 207*f,* 209*f*
Tight contact lens syndrome, 102
Timolol, 263
  for angle closure glaucoma, 137
  for carotid-cavernous sinus
    fistula, 212
  for central/branch retinal artery occlu-
    sion, 175
  for hyphema, 61
  for phacolytic glaucoma, 147
Tobramycin, 264
  for bleb-associated infections, 144
  for corneal abrasion, 49
  for endophthalmitis, 124
Trabecular meshwork, 8, 9*f*
Trabeculectomy, previous, and bleb-
  associated infections, 142, 143*f*
Traction retinal detachment, 167
  with diabetic retinopathy, 168
Trauma, 43–84
  blow-out fractures, 81–84
  chemical and thermal injury, 55–58
  conjunctival and corneal laceration,
    50–54
  corneal abrasion, 46–49
  corneal foreign body, 43–45
  hyphema, 59–61
  intraocular foreign body, 65–67
  lens subluxation or dislocation, 62
  lid laceration, 76–80
  recurrent erosion syndrome, 50
  ruptured globe and scleral
    rupture, 72
Traumatic cataract, 132*f*
Traumatic glaucoma, 138–141
  admission for, 140
  examination findings, 138, 139*f*
  examination outline, 140
  follow up, 140
  grading of hyphema with, 138*t*

Traumatic glaucoma (*Cont.*):
  ICD-9 code for, 140
  treatment, 140
  urgent referral for, 140
Traumatic iritis, 119–121
  examination outline, 119
  follow up, 121
  history, 119
  ICD-9 codes for, 121
  laboratory work up in, 119
  ocular findings, 119, 120*f*
  treatment, 121
Traumatic macular hole, 68–70, 71*f*
Traumatic optic neuropathy, 75
  examination findings, 75
  examination outline, 75
  follow up, 75
  ICD-9 codes for, 75
  treatment, 75
Traumatic retinal damage, 68–70
  examination findings, 68–70, 69*f,* 71*f*
  history, 68
  ICD-9 codes for, 70
  treatment, 70
Travoprost, 263
Triamcinolone, 265
Triazole, 264
Trifluorothymidine, for herpetic keratitis,
  108
Trifluridine, 264
Trimethoprim-polymixin, 264
  for bacterial conjunctivitis, 87
  for dacryocystitis, 204
  for orbital cellulitis, 195
Trimethoprim-sulfamethoxazole, 264
Tropicamide, 265
Trusopt. *See* Dorzolamide

U

Ulcer(s)
  corneal
    with contact lens keratitis and
      infection, 102

Ulcer(s). corneal (*Cont.*):
  with corneal infections, 101
  with exposure keratopathy, 110
  small peripheral, 101
  vision-threatening, 101
  neurotrophic (sterile), with herpetic
    keratitis, 106
Ultrasonography
  in leukocoria (white pupil), 243
  of retinal detachment, 165
  in vitreous hemorrhage, 161
Unoprostone, 263
Urea, 263
Uveitis, 119–124

V

Vancomycin, 264
  for bleb-associated infections, 144
  for endophthalmitis, 124
  for intraocular foreign body, 65
  for orbital cellulitis, 195
Varicella zoster virus infection
  corneal, 100
  keratitis with, 106–108
  preseptal cellulitis with, 190
Vasoconstrictors
  for allergic conjunctivitis, 94
  for orbital cellulitis, 195
Verapamil, for migraine headache
    prophylaxis, 235
Vidarabine (Vira-A), 264
  for herpetic keratitis, 108
Viral conjunctivitis, 88–91
  examination findings, 88, 89*f*–90*f*
  examination outline, 91
  follow up, 91
  history, 88
  ICD-9 codes for, 91
  treatment, 91
Viral medications, 264
Viroptic. *See* Trifluorothymidine
Vision assessment, 15–18
  low vision testing for, 18

Vision assessment (*Cont.*):
  near vision testing for, 15, 18, 19*f*
  pediatric, 237–238, 239*f,* 239*t,* 240*t*
  Snellen test for, 15, 17*f*
Visual acuity, assessment of, 15–18, 16*t*
  low vision testing for, 18
  near vision test for, 15, 18, 19*f*
  pediatric, 237, 238*f,* 239*t*
  Snellen test for, 15, 17*f*
Visual field(s)
  confrontational, 20, 216*t*
  defects/loss, 215
    etiology of, 215, 216*f,* 217*t*
    glaucomatous cupping, 217*f*
    nerve pathways from retina to occipi-
      tal cortex and, 21*f*
    optic pathway lesions and, 22*f,* 216*f*
  testing, 20, 21*f*–22*f,* 215, 216*f,* 217*t*
    Amsler grid for, 258, 259*f*
    pediatric, 237, 239*f*
  types of, 217*t*
Vitrectomy, 166
Vitreous, 1, 2*f,* 10, 155–185
  slit lamp examination of, 30, 31*f*
Vitreous detachment, posterior
  flashes and floaters with, 158
  retinal detachment with, 167
Vitreous hemorrhage, 159–161
  with diabetic retinopathy, 168, 170
  examination findings, 159, 160*f*
  examination outline, 159
  flashes and floaters with, 155–158
  follow up, 161
  history, 159
  ICD-9 code for, 161
  imaging studies in, 161
  laboratory studies in, 161
  with shaken baby syndrome, 254
  treatment, 161
  work up in, 161
Vitritis, 155
Vortex vein, 2*f*
Vossius' ring
  with hyphema, 59, 60*f*
  with lens subluxation or dislocation, 62

W

Watkze-Allen test, 185, 185*t*
Weiss ring, with flashes and floaters, 157
Wet macular degeneration, 180, 181*f*
White blood cells, in anterior chamber.
    See Hypopyon
White pupil (leukocoria), 243–244
  causes of, 244*t*
  examination findings, 243, 245*f*
  examination outline, 243
  follow up, 244
  history, 243
  ICD-9 codes for, 244
  imaging studies in, 243

White pupil (leukocoria) (*Cont.*):
  laboratory tests in, 243
  treatment, 243
  work up, 243
Wood's lamp, in corneal staining, 27

X

Xalatan. *See* Latanoprost

Z

Zonular fibers, 9*f*
Zygomatic bone, 12, 13*f*